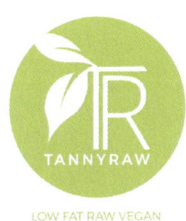

Copyright © 2019, Tanya Murphy

All rights reserved. No part of this book may be reproduced, stored in a retrieval system, or transmitted, in any form or by any means electronic, mechanical, photocopying, recording, or otherwise without the prior written permission of the copyright holder. Printed in the United States of America.

www.TannyRaw.com

ISBN 9781077535084

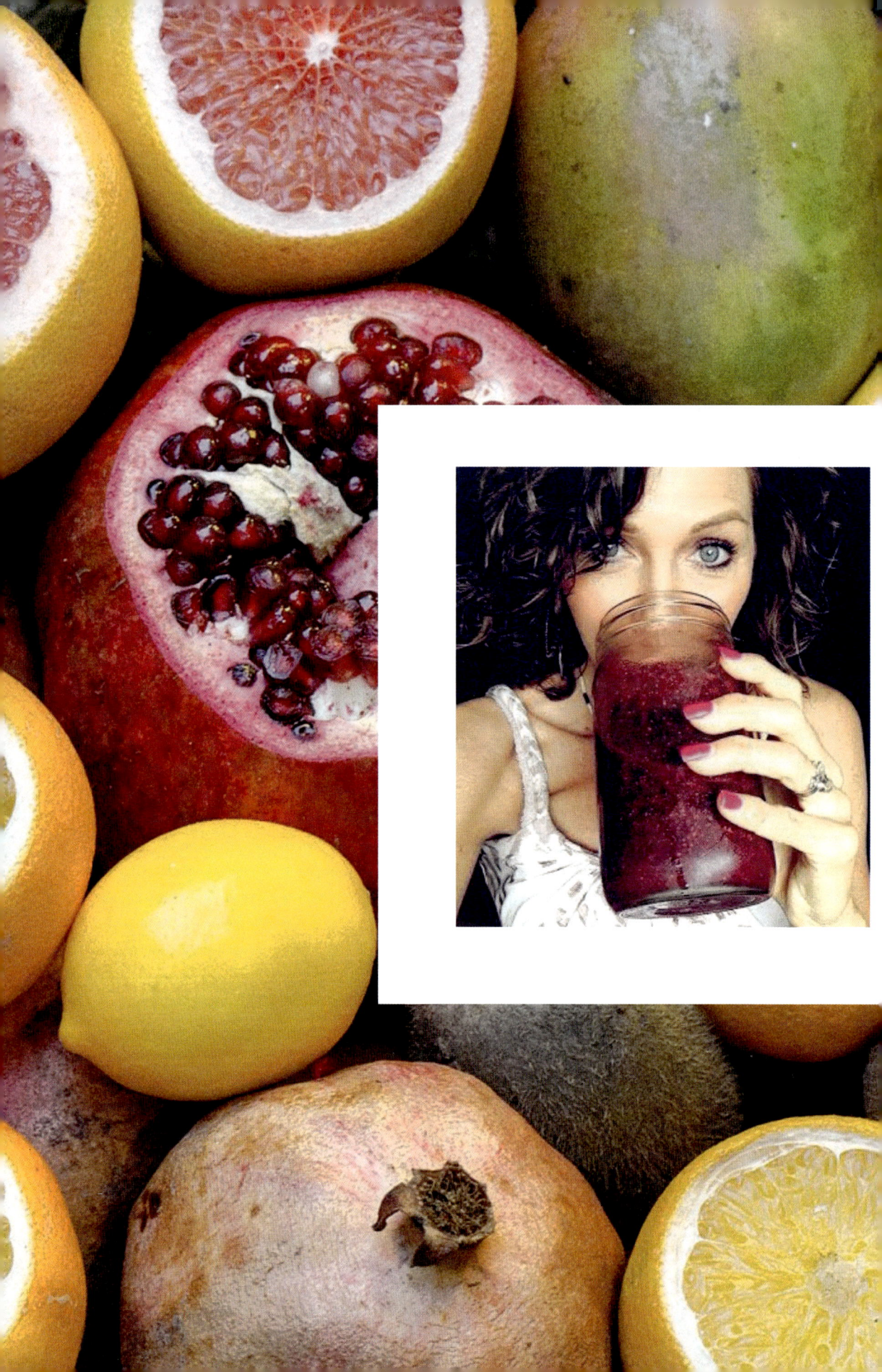

Table Of Contents

Raw Vegan Tips

Intro ... 6

What's Your 'Why'? ... 10

A Plan = Protection ... 14

Journaling ... 18

Food Combining ... 22

Stretch The Fat ... 24

Sprouting ... 28

Intermittent Fasting ... 32

Dealing With Detox ... 36

Recipes

Dips, Soups & Sauces

Cukes & Cream Sauce/Dip ... 42

Nutty Nori Roll Dipping Sauce ... 43

Simple Salsa ... 44

Blood Orange Butterfly Dressing ... 45

Avocado Dip ... 46

Smooth & Savoury Tomato Dip ... 47

My Sweet n' Smooth Dipping Sauce ... 48

Yummy Yellow Squash Dip ... 49

Easy Peasy Dip ... 50

Hearty Carrot Soup ... 51

Simple Slaw ... 52

Savoury Slaw ... 53

Tanny's So Simple Sauce ... 54

Tahini Treat Dipping Sauce ... 55

Creamy Pumpkin Seed Dressing ... 56

Sweet & Zesty Dipping Sauce/Dressing ... 57

On A Coconut Dip Kick ... 58

Hemp Seed Heart Salad Dressing ... 59

Sweet & Spicy Carrot Almond Dressing ... 60

Raw Vegan Sauce With A Kick ... 61

Sweet Almond Dipping Sauce ... 62

Mexican Fiesta Dip ... 63

TannyRaw Fennel Pea Soup ... 64

Walnut Mushroom Soup ... 65

Sweet Sunshine Carrot & Tomato Soup ... 66

Cucumber Avocado Soup ... 67

Detox Elixirs, Tonics & Smoothies

Anti-Inflammatory Brain Booster ... 71

Tummy Tamer ... 71

Mango Crush ... 72

The Clear Cleanser ... 73

Creamy Coconut Smoothie ... 74

Vanilla Peach Smoothie ... 75

Paradise In A Glass Smoothie ... 76

Tropical Storm Smoothie ... 77

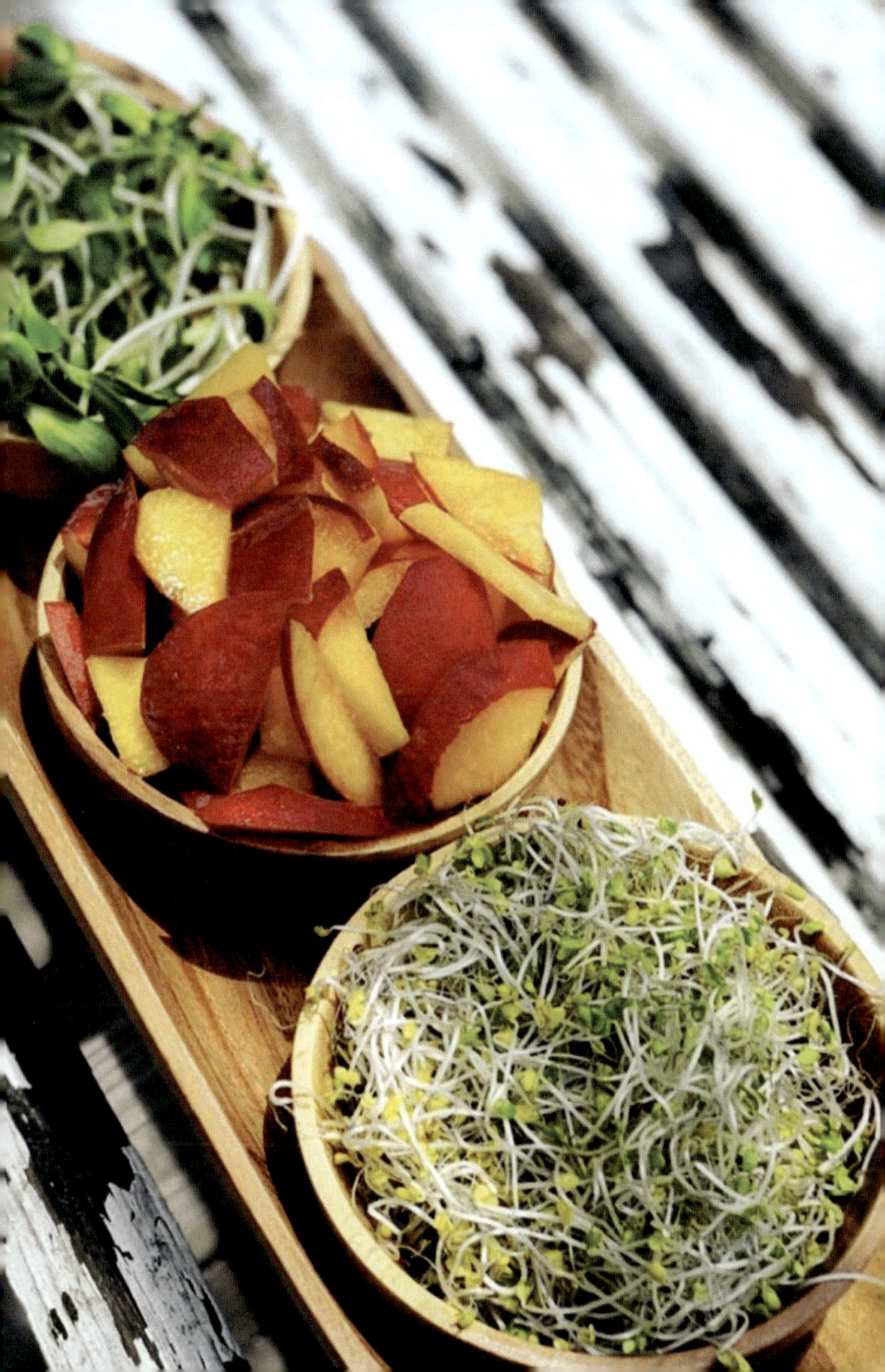

Intro

True vibrant health begins with self-care.

Transformation happens when the pain of remaining the same outweighs the pain of change.

As I aged into my early thirties, I had been diagnosed with Lupus, IBS, leaky gut, nodular acne, brain fog, rheumatoid arthritis, and depression. I was in pain, overwhelmed with my life, broke and somewhere around 209 lbs, I stopped looking at the scale. It was, of course, my measure of success (regardless of how I felt). I could barely move to play with my two young children and everything was just flat out harder than I remembered in my twenties. I knew something was wrong and I didn't know how to fix it. At 29, I was prescribed Methotrexate, Prednisone, and blood infusions because I was in so much pain and so sick. This was my breaking point.

I was so scared of the side effects of the drugs that I wanted to streamline my way to health. It was no longer just about losing weight. It was about surviving. I wanted more and I was so tired of my life skipping beats and going around in circles like a record playing the same old dusty song. And, it finally occurred to me that my relationship with food and how it fueled my body had to change. It was my last hope.

Eighteen years ago, I didn't know where to start and there weren't many resources readily accessible on clean eating. It was all Atkins, Weight Watchers, The Mediterranean Diet—to name a few. The internet was still on the horizon then so I had to look hard for a diet I hadn't tried or someone out there who could explain to me the science behind food as fuel without being too dry and academic.

As I dug deeper after several years on my own, I began to find voices that seemed to be coming from out of the dark—true health advocates like Dr. Doug Graham (author of the 80/10/10 Diet) and Drs. Rick and Karen Dina. My world was opened up to the raw vegan lifestyle nearly a decade

Health is power. All you have to do is take it.

later with the help of these experts. I am so grateful for these masters in the field of nutrition. They were a guiding light in my health journey and continue to inspire me with their impactful messages of healing.

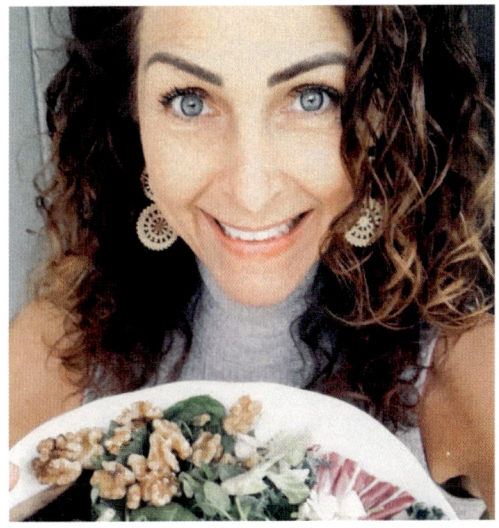

My hope is that you will find some of that support here in this book!

I remember my mantra: "I eat plants. Live food for a live body." I was teaching elementary students at the time and I remember the witching hour—when the cupcakes, or birthday cake, or pot luck would be calling my name to the teachers' lounge at 3 p.m. I would walk past daily and repeat, "I eat plants. Live food for a live body."

Over time, I began to heal and as I did, I was more and more driven by the results. I waffled between stages of having blood sugar issues to overloading on plant fats. It wasn't until I learned about food combining (which I'll get into) that I came to a place where my relationship with food truly transformed.

I didn't have to think about food anymore. Don't get me wrong. Eating became a truly pleasurable experience. My taste-buds changed. With each new combination of flavors I tried, it was like putting on a pair of glasses for the first time and seeing leaves on a tree up close. Because I gave my body time to detox and heal, I became less dependent on eating as a response or habit and more dependent upon what my body was telling me it needed.

It was a game. How could I use food to optimize my healing process? I had benchmarks. My pain disappeared. Over the course of eight months, I lost 88 pounds. My hair began to grow back in. I could play longer with my children. My eyes became brighter and changed color. My vision improved. Doctors told me to keep doing what I was doing.

And for nearly two decades, I stuck to it. There was no magical moment that summed it up. I just continued to find myself as I found my health. Thankfully, I gravitated toward other people trying to get to their best version of themselves. This lifestyle has become easy and effortless for me. It doesn't define me. It refines me.

I want to thank you for picking up this book. It's a big deal for me. It means the world that you would invite me on your path.

This is not a book on dieting. I'm sending this out to you in hopes that it will give you some delicious inspiration and support for beautiful clean raw vegan living. I want to give you all the things I can squeeze into this little book.

I want to show you that you can do this.

Healing is real. Health is power. All you have to do is take it.

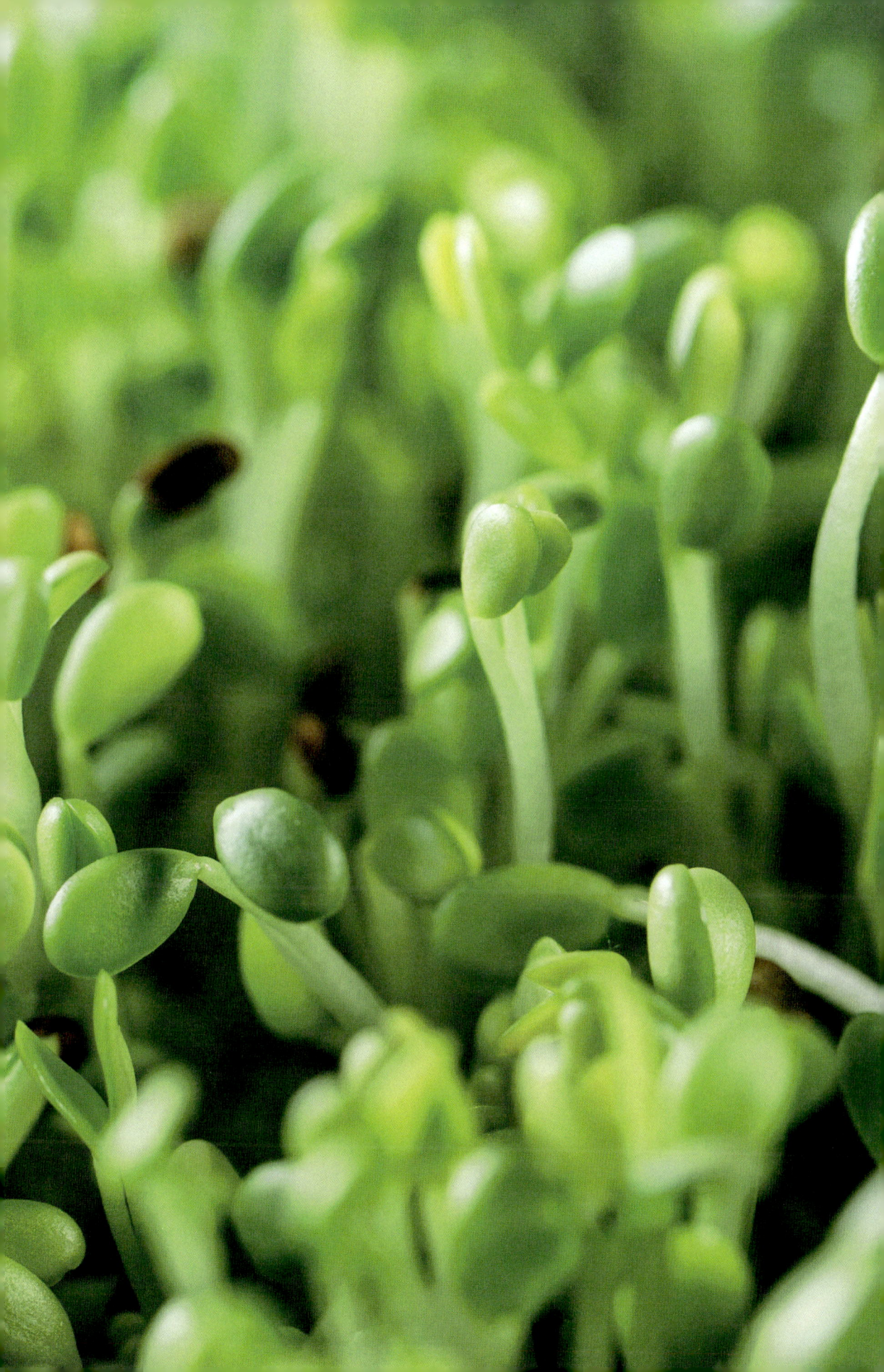

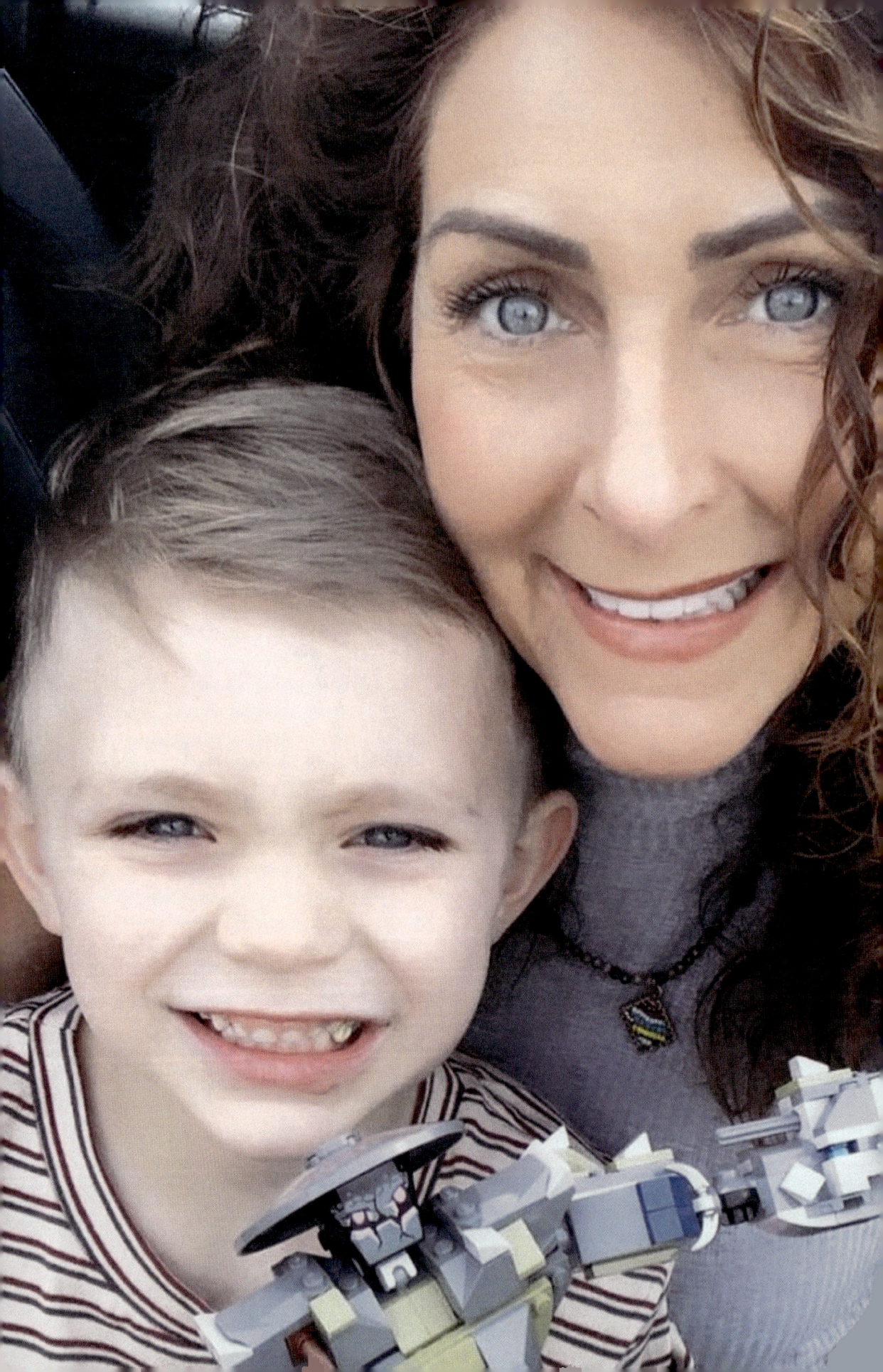

What's Your 'Why'?

It seems like I get the same question (in different forms) almost daily...

How can I make a change in my diet and lifestyle when:

...My family doesn't support me?

...I don't know where to start?

...My cravings always win over?

...I can't afford to eat on a raw vegan diet?

...I travel all the time?

...I'm in the middle of a divorce?

...My health is so bad, it seems like it's too late?

The list goes on. I am not here to say that change is easy, and before I changed my lifestyle and diet to raw vegan, I dealt with many of the issues I listed above. The truth is, I had to hit rock bottom to make the change that brought me to where I am today. Once I hit my breaking point, I had to really think hard about how much control I actually had in my life. Good or bad, out of my control or not, I accepted that it's not about what happens to me, but how I respond that defines me.

I want to spare you rock bottom. I want to show you that change is possible and it is something that is already inside you. You don't have to hit a breaking point to swing the pendulum in a different direction.

I believe you're always one decision away from a totally different life.

We get so wrapped up in these patterns that we forget we can exercise our choice to make change. We can push ourselves and rationalize our way into burnout, but we can't push ourselves into a healthy lifestyle? We have choices, Y'all. We're responsible for our decisions.

I'm here to tell you that if you want to make a shift in your health, your relationships, your mindset, then you must remind yourself continuously that you can change course at any time despite and/or because of the odds working against you.

The one thing that should remain is a strong sense of your 'why'.

In order to achieve change, you must give yourself space and perspective to investigate why you want that shift in your life. Why does it mean so much to you? Dig deep and be real with yourself.

You have to fight for that why and continuously remind yourself that it's worth every obstacle that comes your way. Your why will motivate you and lead you to solutions that come from within.

It feels very different to focus on what you do want as opposed to complaining and feeling bad about what you don't want. What does it look like on the other side where true health lives, where relationships prosper, and life becomes more manageable because you're feeling better than ever? What does it feel like? Know this before you ever even make that first step. This will then be associated with your why, which is just the motivation you need.

Show up for yourself. You show up for others all the time. Rather than focusing on where you were and why I want you to move your attention to the present moment and be the change you wish to see in yourself. Be it. Show up and say, "Here I am." I promise you, the more you act the part and make small decisions that snowball into big changes, the more you feel it — and it's real, Y'all.

Think about it. We've dealt with change throughout our lives and somehow we've survived each one, good and bad. Births, deaths, marriages, divorces— through the most joyful and painful moments in life, we move forward.

You can choose health. You can do this.

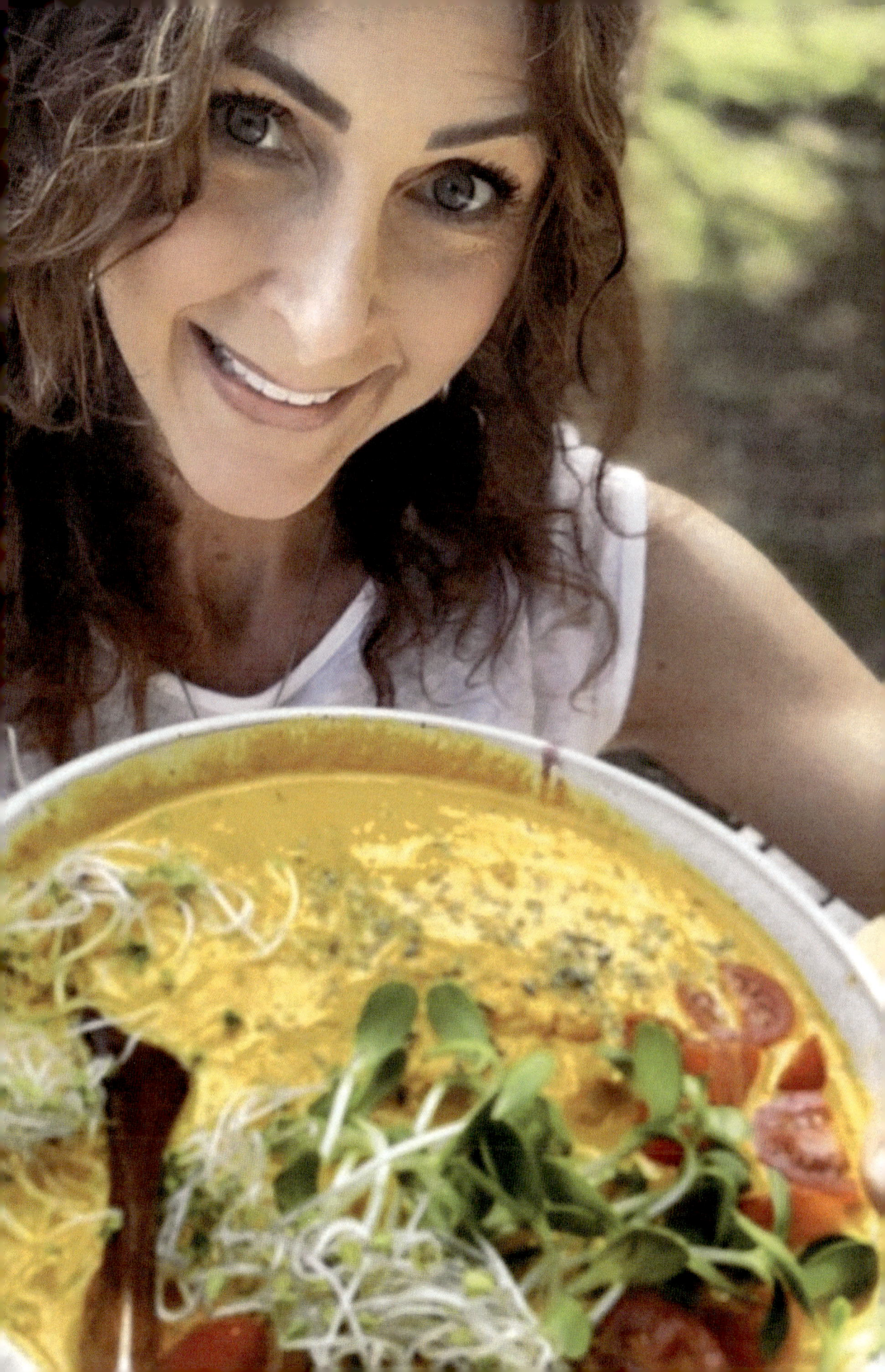

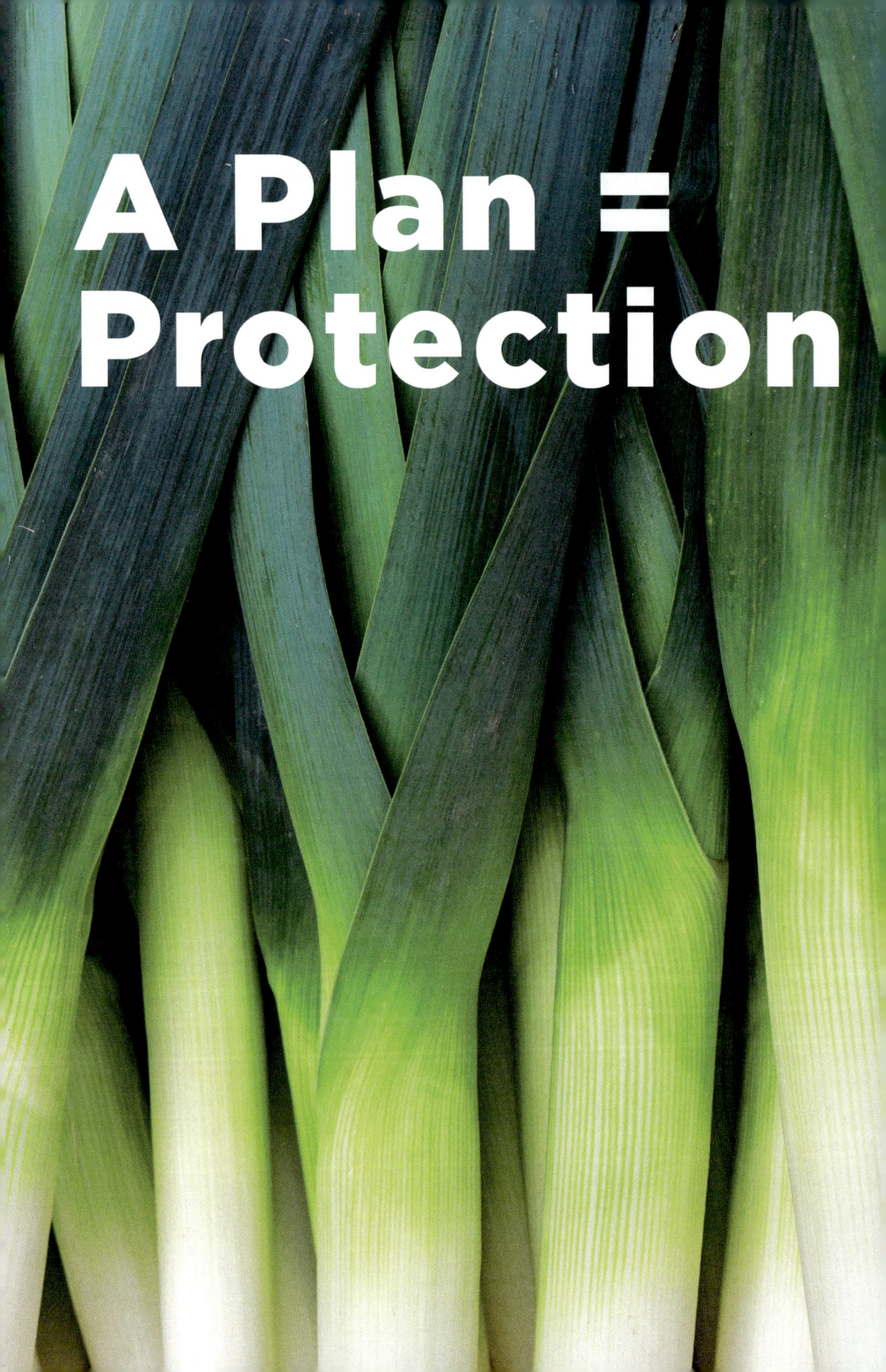

Do Different. Get Different.

We all have a default mode. During times of joy, crisis, celebration, mourning—you name it—we have our own coping skills. For some, it's forgetting to feed the body during these periods. For many, we eat our way through emotions.

Here's the thing. These are moments in our lives that we can always expect no matter how unexpected they feel. So, you have to do different to get different. And once you discover how to overcome your default mode, you can create your plan and leave yourself options.

Keep it simple.

Whether you're in the moment and facing a challenge head-on or you're anticipating how a BBQ crowd will respond to your snap peas and zoodles—do not become overwhelmed. At that moment—whatever it is that you're fixing to choose—choose differently, move into action.

I want you to master this moment without the complication of over-thinking each scenario.

So, I've broken down what a simple raw vegan plan could look like:

A liquid in the am. (celery juice or lemon water)

Smoothie (or chew the ingredients)

And another Smoothie (or chew the ingredients)

Snack (your required amount of fruit balanced with something green)

Simple Dinner (A base of greens, taking your amount of fat, stretching it out into a raw vegan dressing, a soup, or a sauce. Add your seaweed and other veggies.)

It's really that simple.

I also wanted to add this nugget of wisdom:

Hungry is not an emergency.

One of my Raw Resetters famously said those words. I love them. Always be prepared.

Here's how it works:

Here's an exercise I want you to do today.

Make a list of your known triggers.

Create an if/then statement for each trigger.

If _____ (this happens), then I will _____ (take this action).

If I am running errands with my toddler, then I will always have an apple and crunchy veggie crackers—some kind of fresh snack—in my bag before I leave the house.

It's not difficult. It's just different.

If I go out to eat, then I am going to order a salad and veggies and, if possible, have avocado diced on top with lemons squeezed for the dressing.

If I get into a conflict with a co-worker, then I will take a walk around the parking lot to cool off (not run to the vending machine).

If we are unable to predict how we will act in {blank} situation, we leave ourselves unarmed without a plan leaving us in default mode—something that hasn't worked many times over.

How do we prepare for the messy stuff and prevent going "off the wagon?"

Have a plan.

What happens when you're making dinner for your family and you start reminiscing about the good old days of cooked food? **Have a plan.**

Your cousin calls and invites you over for one of her awesome picnic pool parties, but you're worried you'll be tempted by the pot-luck. **Have a plan.**

When you have a plan, you have protection. And you can go anywhere and you can do anything.

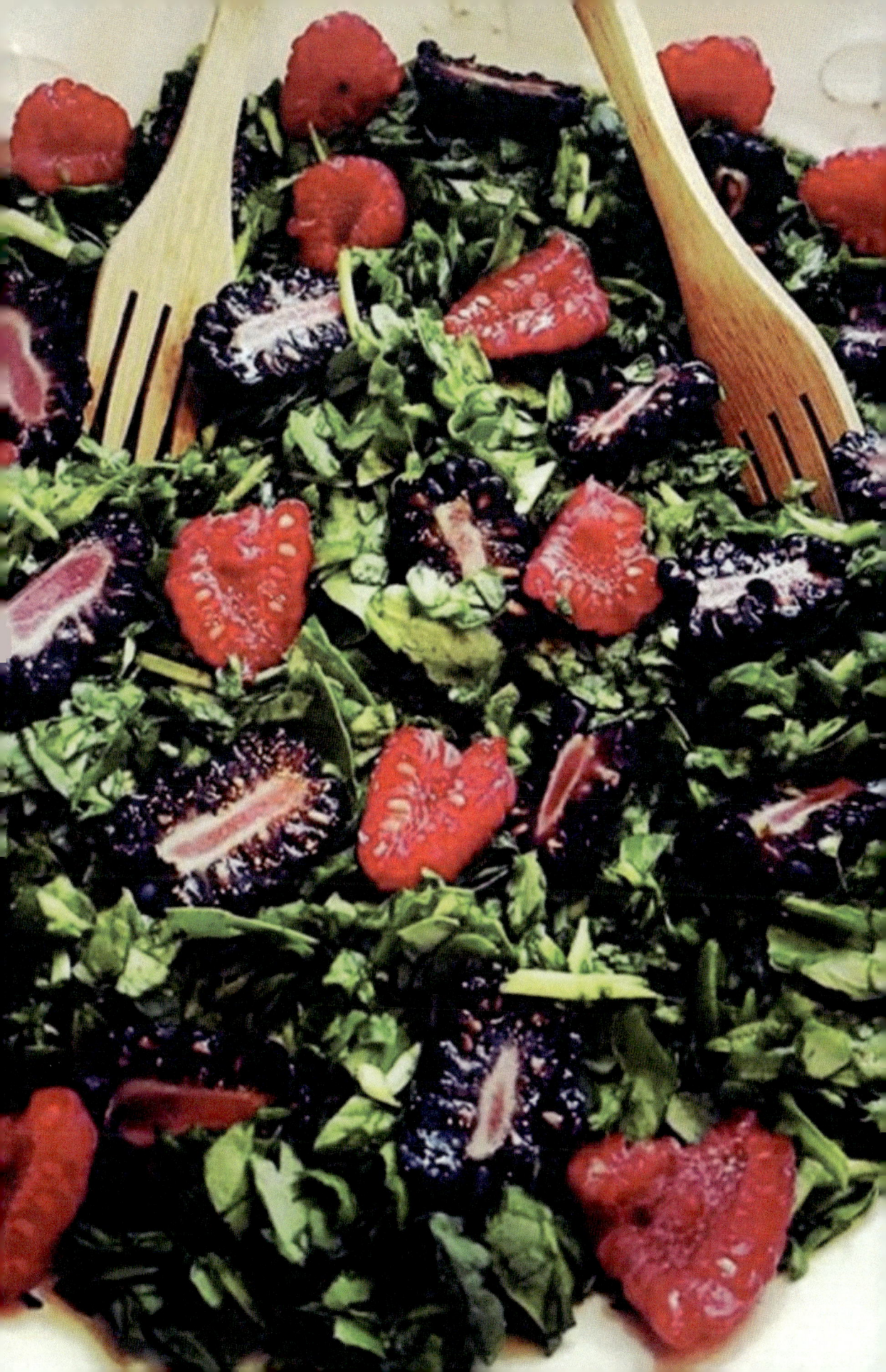

Journaling

Don't try to be perfect. Just try to be better than yesterday.

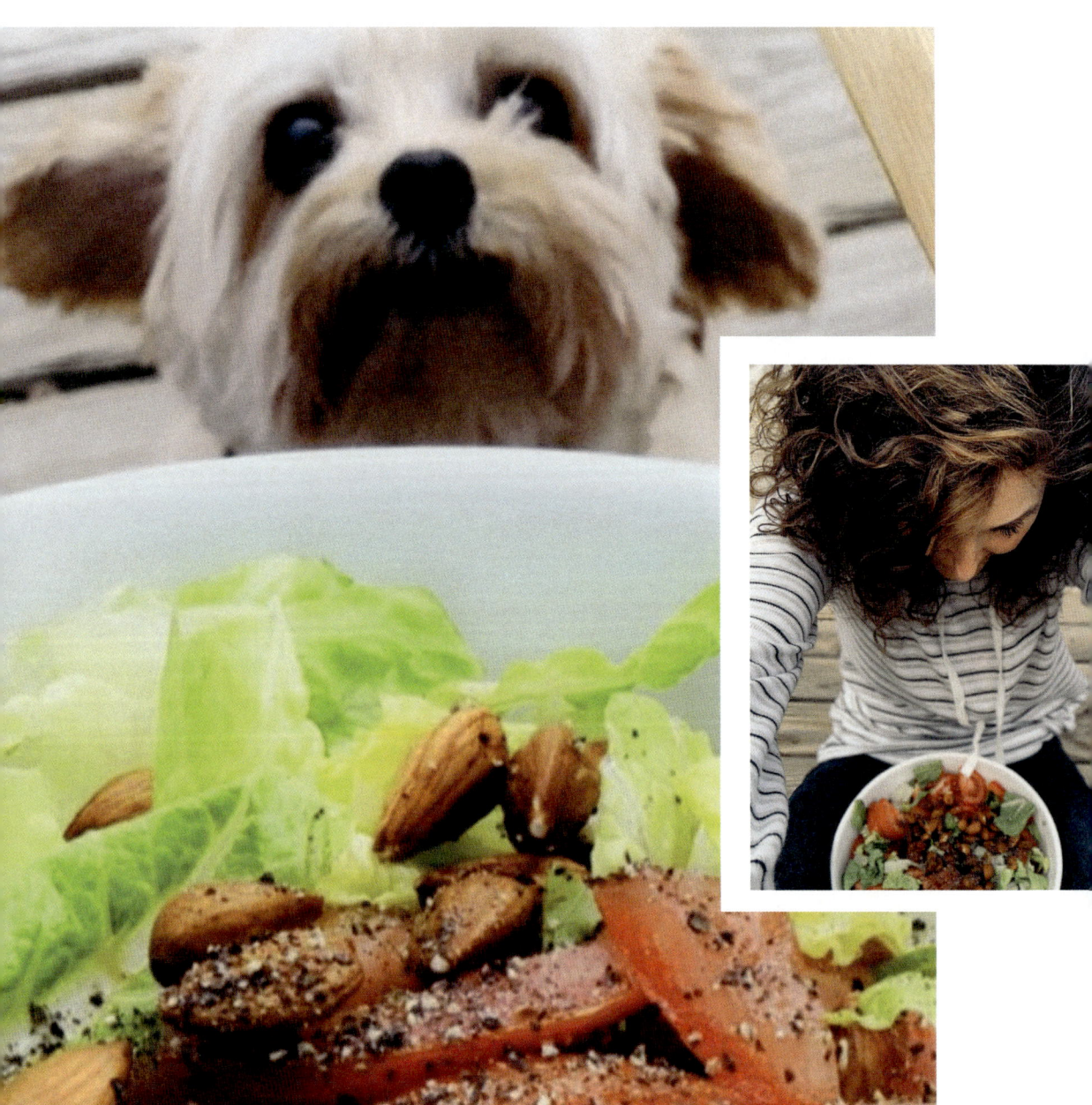

Begin a journal. This should be a special journal that you keep close at hand and use to document your habits, meals, and other significant events that impacted your decision making that day. I'm not asking you to pour all of your deep dark secrets into a book and keep a lock on it. I'm telling you that if you track your habits on a day-to-day basis, as those pages accumulate, you will see patterns, where these patterns are interrupted, and if your results are in alignment with the decisions you are making every day.

Do this as you're sipping your tea at night. Or, find a time during lunch to reflect and keep tabs. Just keep that journal near because it will serve as a guide and help keep your plan in action.

Get a special bound journal—one you can't tear the pages out of. Make sure it's beautiful and sings to you so that you're drawn to it daily.

You can track whatever it is that is important to you, but I thought I would include a guide if you're looking for a place to start. Consider the following when you track your day:

Did you drink your water?

Did you have your greens?

Did you space dinner and bedtime?

Did you have your tea? What kind? Why not?

Did you have a bowel movement today?

Was something different in your diet? Document this.

Another thing to consider is tracking the following for meal specific journaling:

How much: List the amount of the food/drink item. This might be measured in volume (1/2 cup), weight (2 ounces), or the number of items (12 celery stalks).

What kind: Write down the type of food/drink. Be as specific as you can. Don't forget to write down extras, such as toppings, sauces, or dressings.

When: Keep track of the time of day you eat.

Where: Make note of where you eat. If you are at home, write down the room. For instance, at the dining room table, in the kitchen, or on the sofa. If you are out, write down the name of the restaurant or if you are in the car.

With Whom: If you eat by yourself, write "alone." If you are with friends or family members, list them.

Activity: In this column, list any activities you do while you eat. You could be working, watching TV, or playing a game.

Mood: Chart your mood throughout your day. When do you have the most energy? When do you feel like you've had enough?

It's really about what works for you. So, find 10 minutes out of your day to jot down all of the things you want to document and start tracking today.

My most important advice on journaling: Don't aim to be perfect. Do not tear out any pages or scribble out any blips. These are challenges that ultimately become victories once you get yourself back on track. And you will.

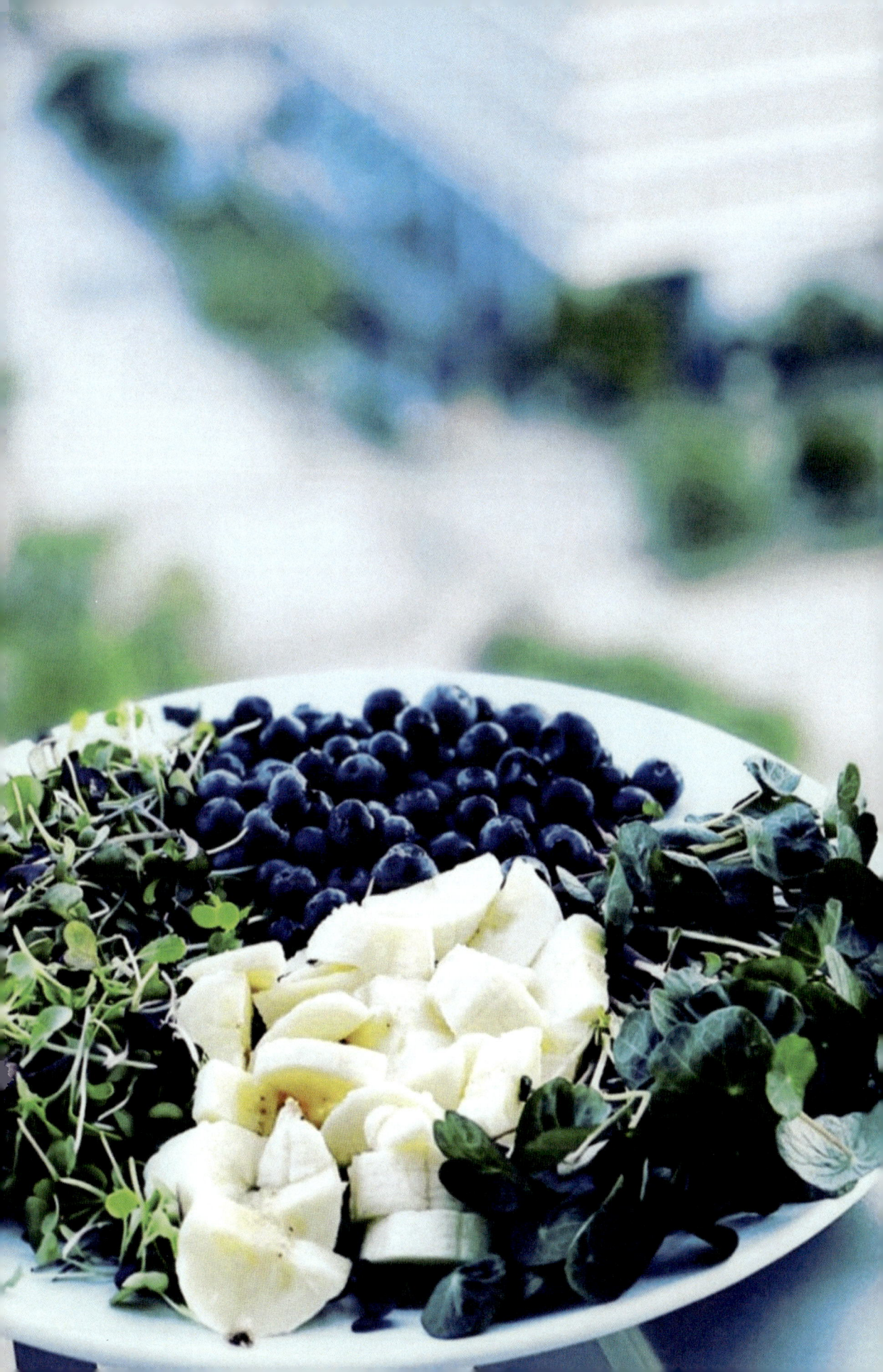

Food Combining

Aim to get as many power-packed nutrients per forkful as possible.

Y'all, once I learned the concept of food combining, the game changed. It was a process that took some time as I tested combinations and journaled my body's response, but with each new discovery came new gains that only continue to surprise me.

I experienced less and less bloat to a point of having a flat belly around the clock. My energy sky-rocketed and sustained itself throughout the day. The mental fog disappeared. I learned how to count on my body, knowing how it would react to certain foods and combos—not to mention the world around me.

This process is different for everyone, but once you start to get the hang of it, the benefits are massive.

Different foods digest at different rates. In essence, I have found that it is impactful to consume the foods that digest fastest to slowest, but also in the right combination based on some simple rules of thumb. Ultimately, we want to avoid fermentation in the stomach. This rotting is at the core of how bacteria, yeast, and fungi develop, causing painful intestinal aches and bloat.

Here's an example: Typically, a food like avocado will take hours to digest, whereas a melon will take about 30 minutes. If I were to eat an avocado (a fat) and wash it down with a juicy cantaloupe...well, Houston, we have a problem. It boils down to chemistry.

I put together a quick chart of foods that combine well and other combinations to avoid. Just remember this: Greens go with EVERYTHING. While fruits will give you that high flying feeling and energy, greens are the engine that keeps the plane flying! Balance is essential!

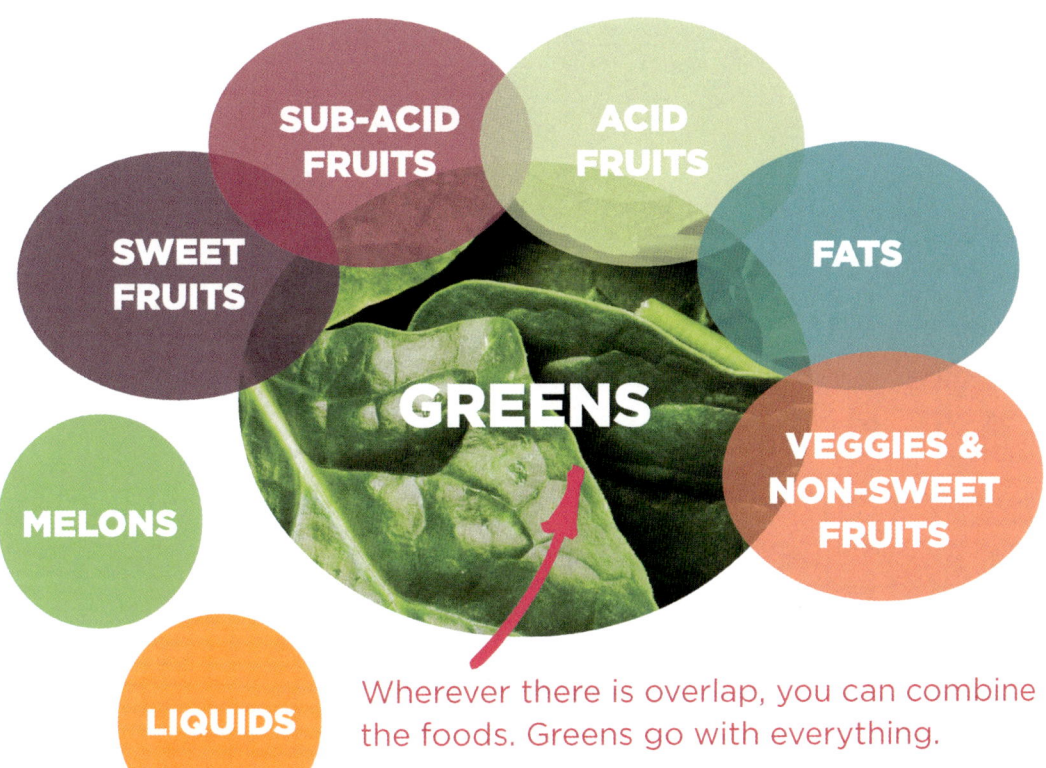

Wherever there is overlap, you can combine the foods. Greens go with everything.

GREENS
- Spinach
- Lettuce
- Kale
- Cilantro
- Collards
- Parsley
- Arugula

ACID FRUIT
- Oranges
- Pineapple
- Lemons
- Blueberries
- Limes
- Grapefruit
- Tomatoes

VEGGIE/NON-SWEET FRUIT
- Cucumber
- Bell Peppers
- Celery
- Squash
- Zucchini
- Starches

SUB-ACID FRUIT
- Apple
- Kiwi
- Cherry
- Grapes
- Blackberries
- Raspberries
- Pear

SWEET FRUIT
- Bananas
- Dates
- Figs
- Persimmon
- Plantain
- Dried Fruit
- Durian

FATS
- Avocado
- Nuts
- Coconut
- Raw Hulled Hemp Seed Hearts
- Flax Seeds

MELONS
- Watermelon
- Cantaloupe
- Honeydew
- Musk melon

Stretch the Fat

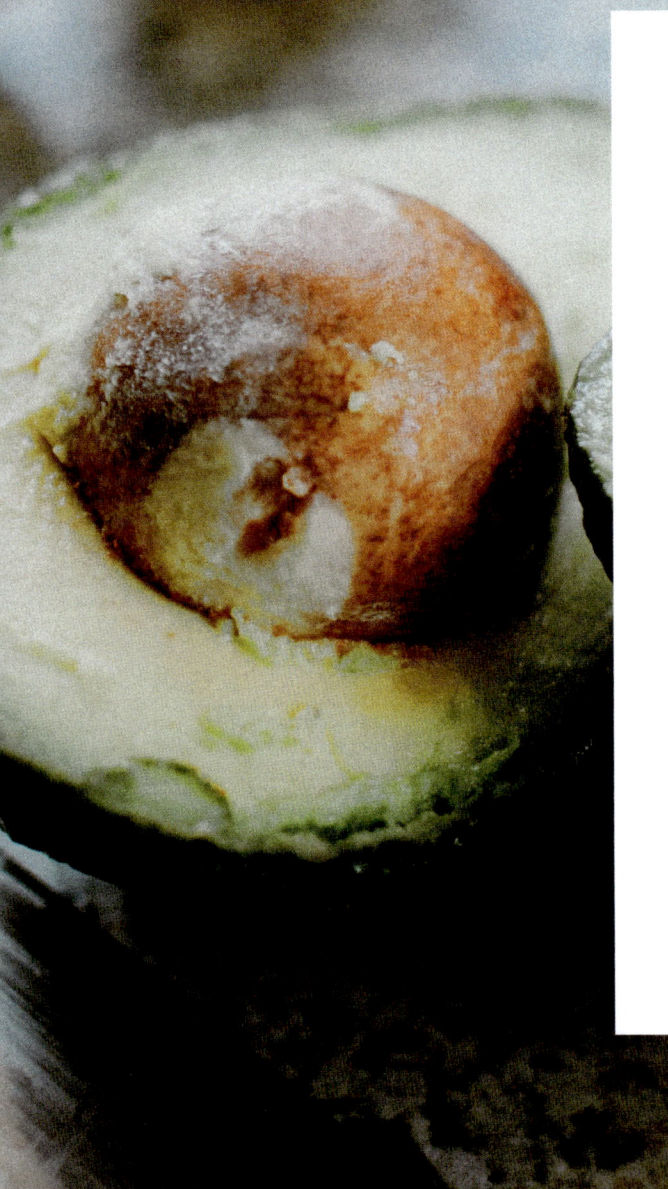

We have to be mindful in our diet of how much fat we're getting. Foods like avocado and nuts are just fine to incorporate into your diet; however, these are not "free" fats. If you're focusing on fats and not getting enough calories from fruit, greens, and veggies, your body is going to get calories from somewhere and that will end up being from the richer fatty foods. To be sure you're striking a balance in terms of fats and calories, I suggest stretching the fat. What I mean by this is that you can use a number of different ingredients to maximize the flavor, create more food, expand the nutritional value, and get more bang for your buck.

Feeding yourself well is the greatest form of self love.

The best way to stretch the fat is by creating a dressing, dip, sauce, or soup. You can literally move from one to the other just by adding different ingredients (therefore, controlling the fat intake and how well the body digests). The most important thing is the meal retains and gains even more nutrients as you transform flavors with key ingredients.

While there is a similar chart in my guide *Dressing For Any Occasion*, I thought I would also include it here as a complement to this book. I think it's handy to have when you're looking for a basic guide to stretching the fat.

Note: When I make these in my high-speed blender, I end up using about half the pitcher for the day. This means I'm getting enough satiation from the balance of fats and fruits—full of flavor, I'm saving money and my meals are planned out for the next day.

Whether you're craving a rich, creamy dressing, a savoury sauce or a hearty dip, there are very simple yet delicious ingredients to help achieve just the right flavor, texture and density while stretching the fats according to your specific needs.

ADDING HEALTHY FATS

1 TBS raw hulled hemp-seed hearts

¼ c fresh ground flax seeds

2 TBS raw nut butter

2 TBS tahini seed butter

½ medium avocado

ADDING VOLUME & FLAVOR WITHOUT ADDING FAT

FOR BASIC VOLUME

1 c celery

1 c peeled zucchini

1 c white button mushrooms

1 c Roma tomatoes

ADDING 'SALT'

1 TBS wakame seaweed

1 TBS dulse flakes

1 TBS kelp flakes

ADDING SWEETNESS

2 TBS lucuma powder

3 dried unsulfured apricots

2—3 dates

½ c sun-dried tomatoes

ADDING ACID

½—1 lemon, peeled

½—1 lime, peeled

¼ raw apple cider vinegar

½ c fresh orange juice

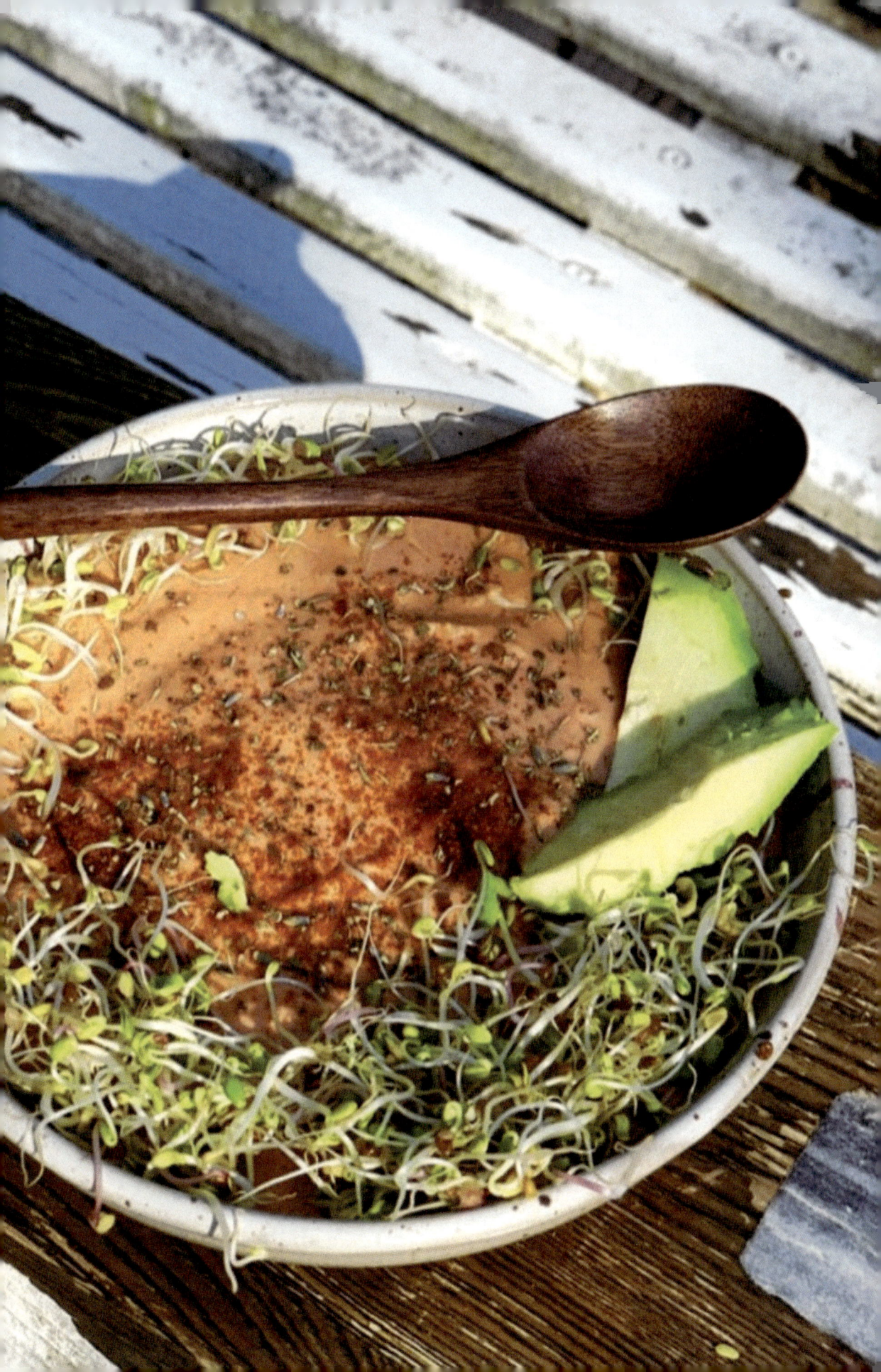

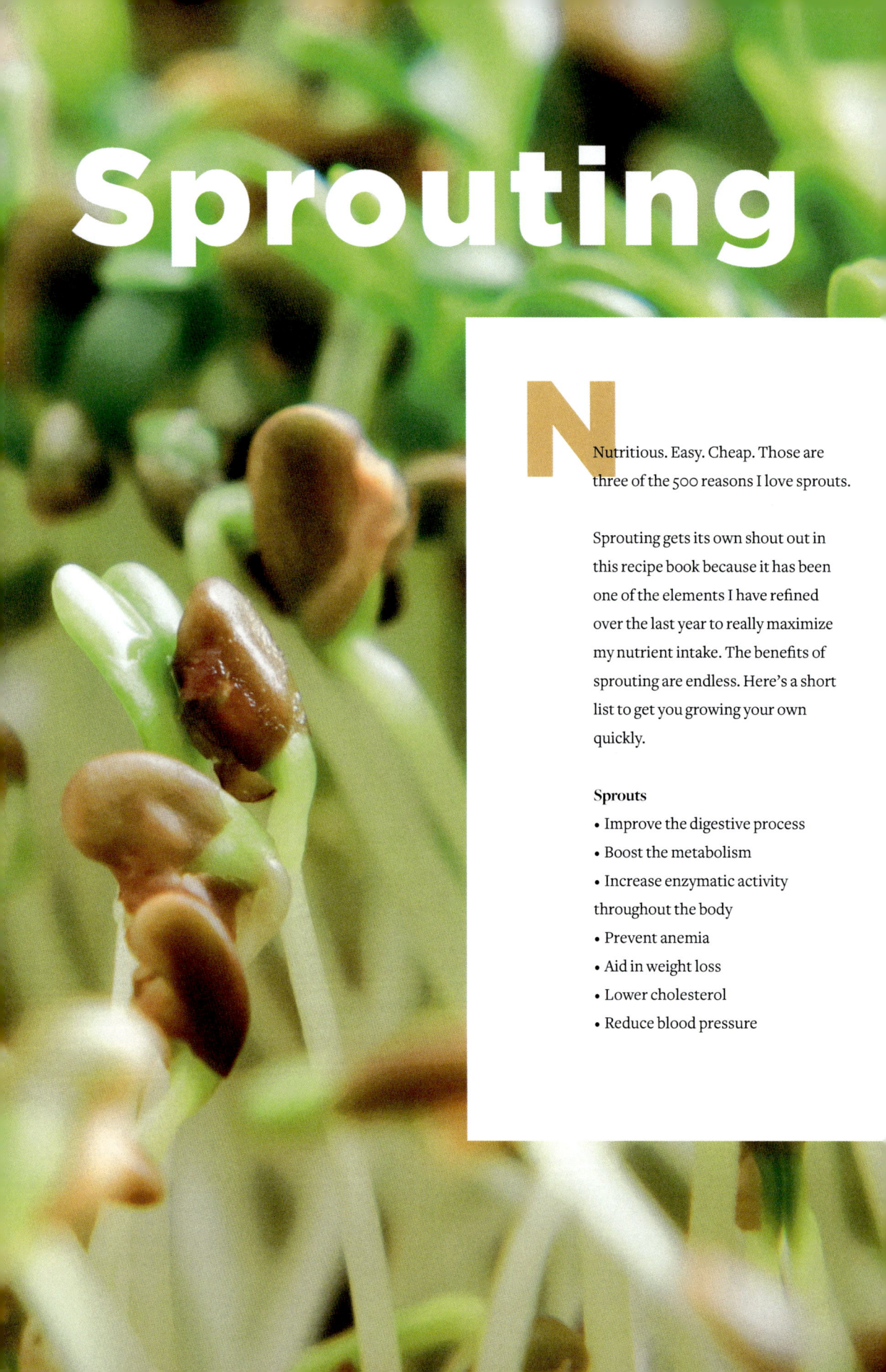

Sprouting

Nutritious. Easy. Cheap. Those are three of the 500 reasons I love sprouts.

Sprouting gets its own shout out in this recipe book because it has been one of the elements I have refined over the last year to really maximize my nutrient intake. The benefits of sprouting are endless. Here's a short list to get you growing your own quickly.

Sprouts
- Improve the digestive process
- Boost the metabolism
- Increase enzymatic activity throughout the body
- Prevent anemia
- Aid in weight loss
- Lower cholesterol
- Reduce blood pressure

Live food for a live body.

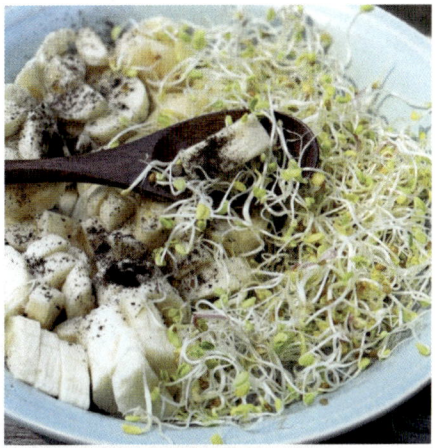

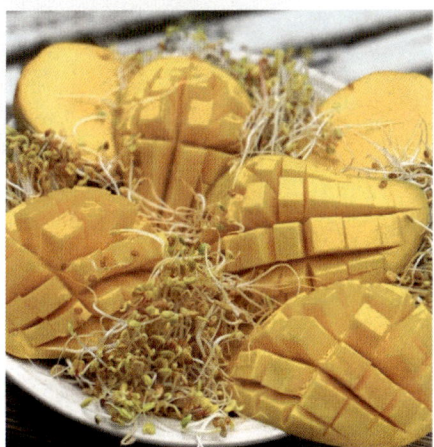

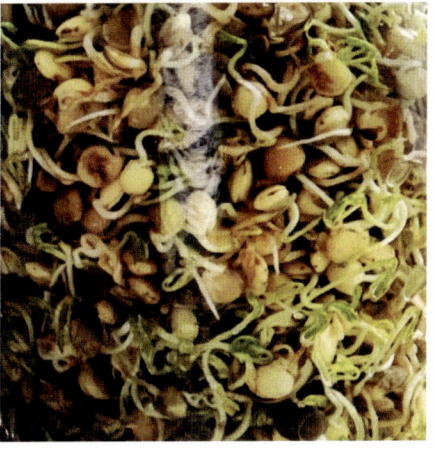

- Prevent neural tube defects in infants
- Boost skin health
- Improve vision
- Support the immune system
- Increase usable energy reserves.

The reason that so many people turn to sprouts as a source of food is that they represent a significantly higher amount of vitamins and nutrients than they do in an un-sprouted form. Typically, a week after sprouting, the sprouts will have the highest concentration and bioavailability of nutrients. Beans must contain a packed storehouse of all the important nutrients that a plant will need to grow in its initial days, so those tiny caps are filled with important organic compounds, vitamins, and minerals that our body can also utilize.

How to grow them at home

This is where it gets fun. It's like a little game. How fast will they grow? After 3 days and a couple of hours, a handful of mung beans sprout into a harvestable nutrient powerhouse for pennies on the dollar.

There are two ways I have sprouted: in a mason jar and a little screen or with an electric device. I use either depending on the mood or how quickly I need them.

If I'm using a mason jar, I generally soak the beans for about 20 hours, drain and rinse them, and then add the moist mung beans to the jar. As they grow, you want to rinse them twice daily.

If you're using an automatic sprouter, I'd follow the directions based on your machine. Generally, you fill it with water to a baseline, add rinsed mung beans to the tray (no need to soak before) and let the water flow. Rise and drain twice a day.

They last about 5 days when rinsed and stored in an air-tight container (once cut).

Types of sprouts include:
Alfalfa (and alfalfa mixtures), Adzuki, baby mung, lentils, and chickpeas, but there are countless more!

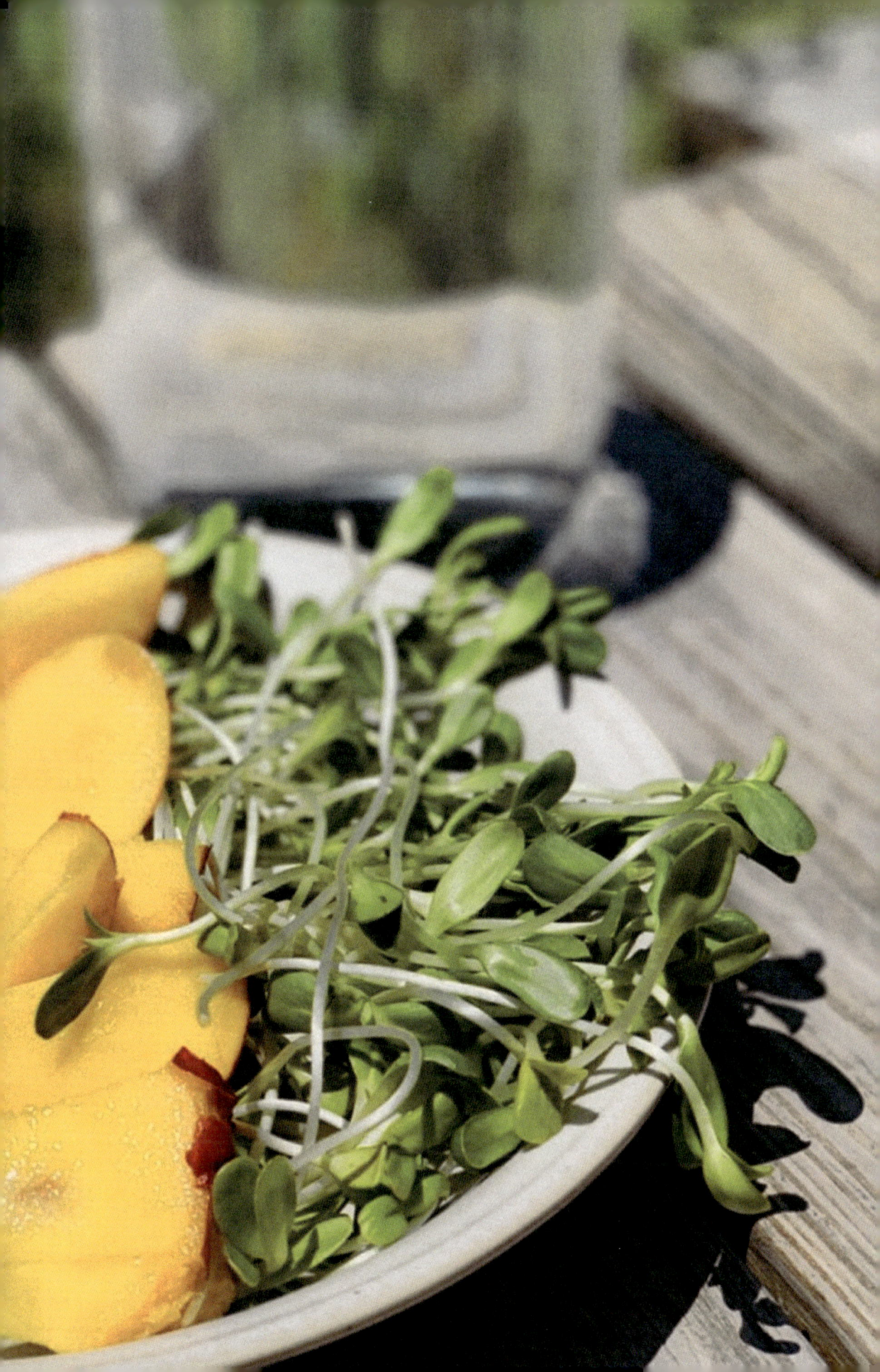

Intermittent Fasting

The best of all medicine is resting and fasting.
—Benjamin Franklin

Y'all, don't run when you see the word "fasting." I'm going to give you a few reasons to consider intermittent fasting, a type of fasting anyone can do, to improve your overall health. I am not talking about food deprivation. I am not talking about fad cleanses that require you starve yourself. No juicing needed here. I'm talking about consuming the same amount of calories and food that you currently eat on a healthy raw vegan plan, but only eating these calories between a shorter window of time.

How does this work? I eat breakfast no earlier than 10 a.m. and I end my meals with dinner at 5:30 p.m. When I do this, any time I spend not eating outside of that window, my body is working to digest the food from earlier and rejuvenate my cells so that I am light and bright for the next day. You give your body everything, including the time it needs within that shorter time frame and it gives back tenfold.

In my own experience, if I am forced to eat any later than 7 p.m., my sleep suffers. I wake up groggy and swollen and lack energy during the day.

Here are some benefits to intermittent fasting according to a number of studies:

Intermittent Fasting helps burn fat.

The journal *Cell Research* published a study that found that after 16 weeks of intermittent fasting, it was shown to prevent obesity. The benefits began to show up around week six. The research also shows that this type of fasting can boost metabolism and help burn more fat—particularly around the belly.

Intermittent Fasting boosts brain power.

According to a number of studies, many doctors and scientists contend that intermittent fasting can promote healthy brain function. In turn, many believe this type of fasting can help prevent diseases like Parkinson and Alzheimer. When you forgo food, your brain is challenged—it needs to find food. This means it kicks into high gear in order to take preventative measures against diseases. During the fasting period—16 hours based on my example—your body is burning fat which produces ketones. These are a major source of energy-boosting brain power.

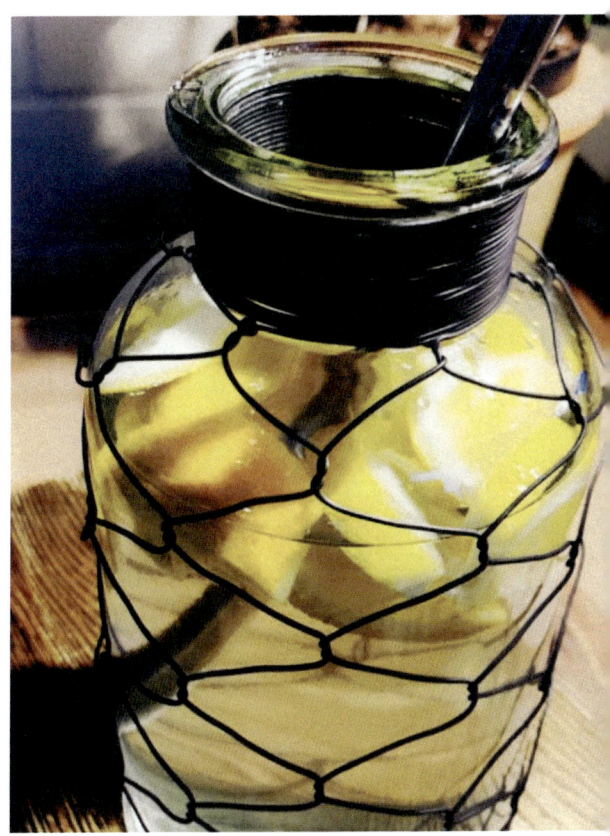

My friend, why wouldn't we want to live lucidly in our lives of love and light? Your life is worth remembering. And if you're feeding your body the right plant foods, why not get more regimented with your eating schedule?

Some studies show that Intermittent Fasting helps prevent diabetes.

Intermittent fasting encourages the body to produce less insulin which may help those who are pre-diabetic. This insulin is also what causes fat to store around the belly. It seems more studies must be done to prove this; however, with all the other benefits listed here, why wouldn't you try this?

Think of an infected hangnail. It's ugly, painful, and sometimes carries puss. It's at risk of getting worse

Intermittent Fasting can help reduce inflammation in the body.

if you don't rinse it, treat it, and reduce the inflammation until it heals. Your body is like one big hangnail on the inside if you're eating nasty processed foods at all hours of the night. Chronic inflammation causes dis-ease and can eventually lead to weight gain. Intermittent fasting can help reduce this inflammation phenomenon. This means less pain in the body, less swelling, smoother, softer skin, and a healthy outward appearance.

Now, if you are considering intermittent fasting, I would definitely recommend speaking to your doctor. We all have our own specific set of circumstances. According to many sources, it is not recommended for those with eating disorders, body dysmorphia, people with type 1 diabetes, and women who are pregnant or breastfeeding. Certain prescriptions can also negatively affect your experience.

So, get all your ducks in a row and give your body some rejuvenating benefits with intermittent fasting if you decide this is right for you.

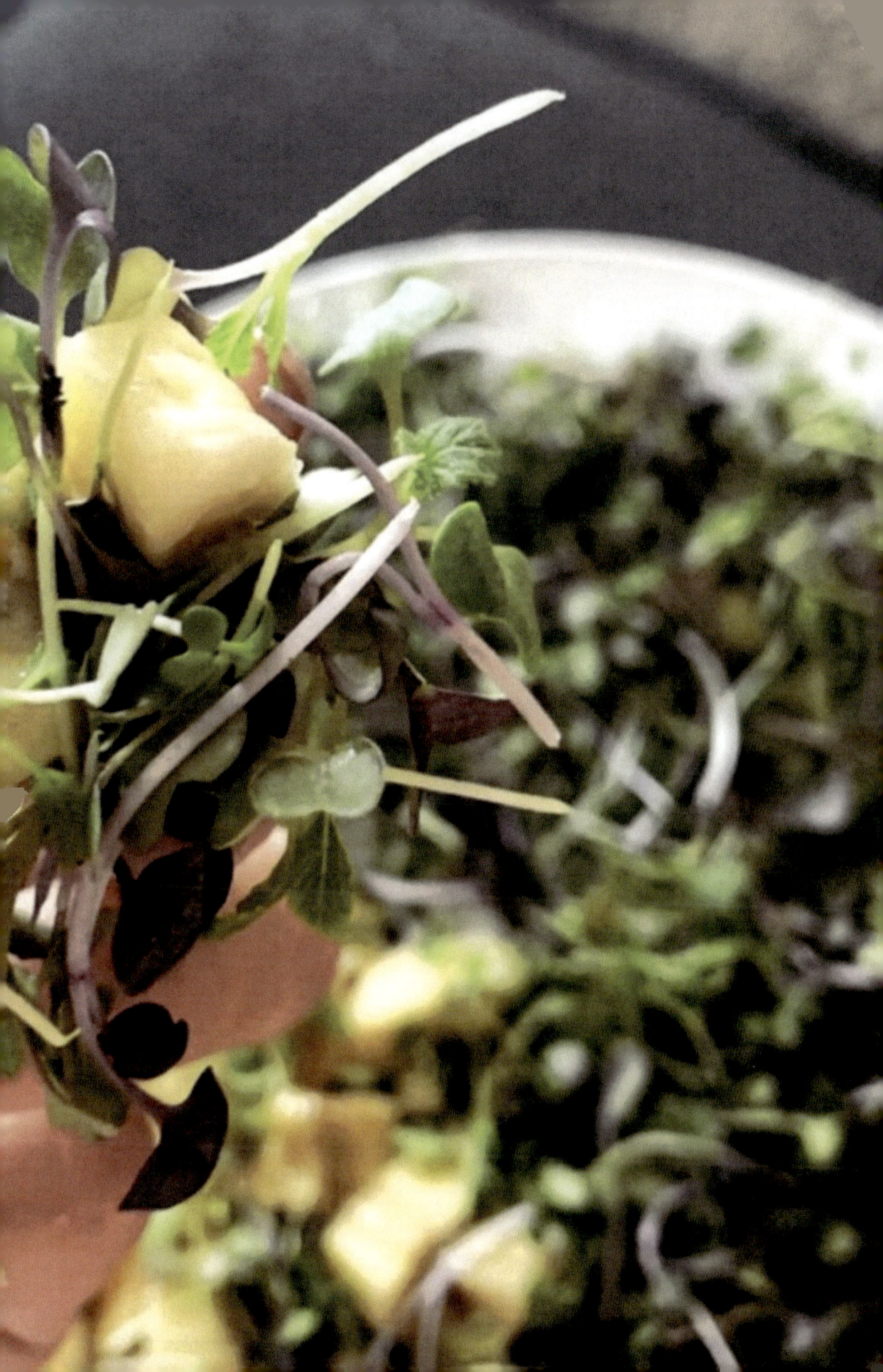

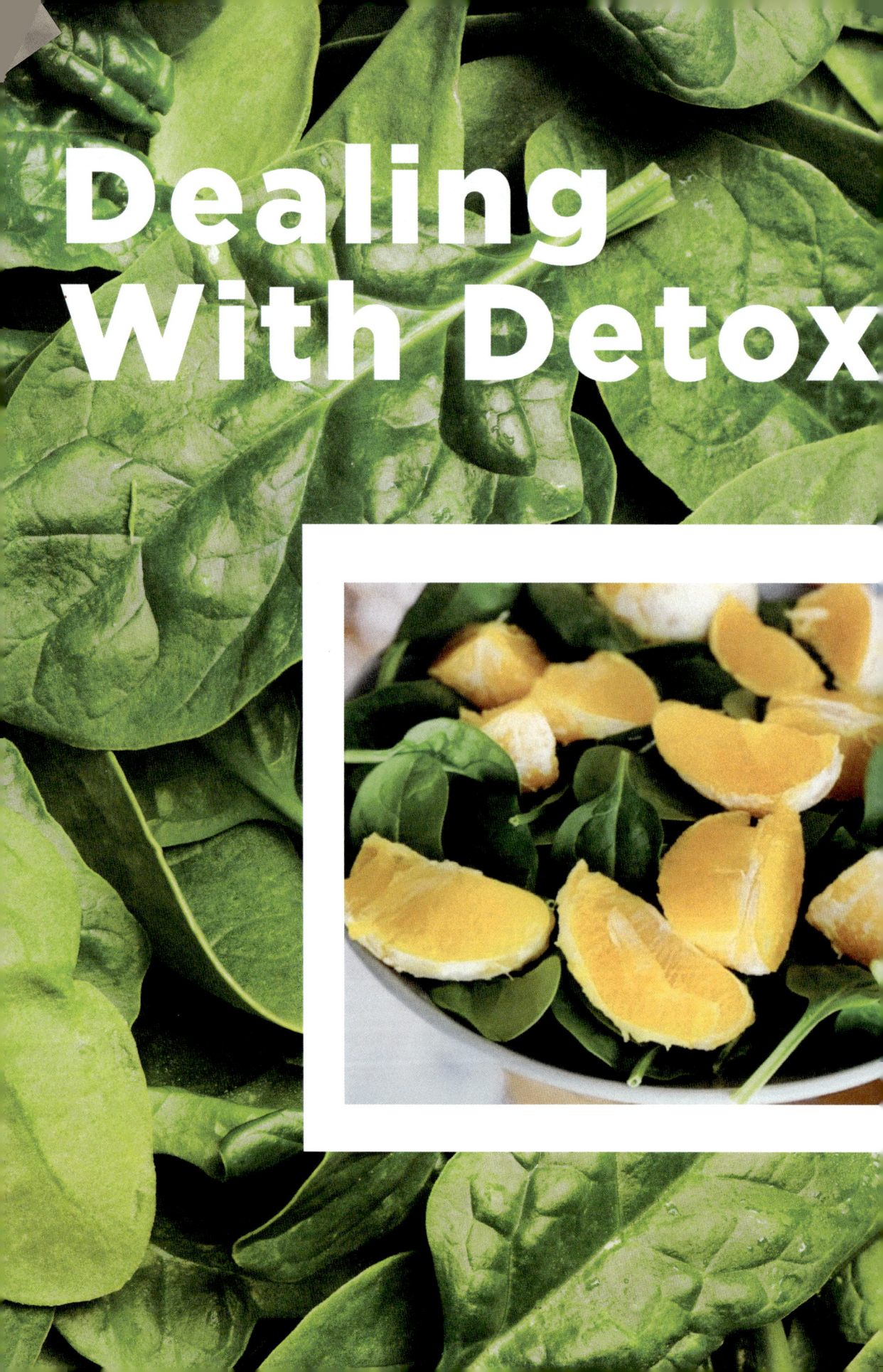

If you're living in the modern world—which you are—You are subject to hundreds of thousands of chemicals and toxins throughout your life. Whole, raw foods are essential to feeling on top of the world and living a truly healthy life; however, when you're moving from a cheeseburger a day to a plant-based diet (or even if you're transitioning from vegan to raw), it is realistic to expect you'll experience some detox symptoms. But don't let that stop you!

Detox, or the fear of it, can keep a lot of people from moving forward with a healthy whole-food raw diet. In so many cases, people begin to cleanse with great intentions, but as symptoms start to show their ugly heads, they turn back rather than move through to the other side.

Our bodies are made up of organs and systems to help us clean up and heal; however, consider how much you accumulate after 10, 20, 30, and 40+ years of eating a standard diet—a diet that's mostly comprised of chemicals, artificial flavors, animal fats, and other junk. These poor organs and systems get bogged down and need a jump start to get back to cleaning house. Think of what happens to a car if you give it the wrong kind of fuel or never change the oil. You can't blame that car for stalling out, right?

Just like our cars, we need maintenance and upkeep. The organs get completely overwhelmed and can shut down.

With all that build-up, our organs and systems get sluggish. The health of our eliminatory organs is actually a huge factor when it comes to getting both healthy and slim. When those things are backed up, there is going to be a struggle.

The Body During Detox

So, a lot of people ask me what's happening to the body during detox. All these toxins that landed in our systems over time can be stored as fat cells. This is the body's way of trying to fight the toxins and protect itself. These fat cells keep the toxins away from your organs, but, as we know, too many fat cells can lead to a host of other issues.

Now, a lot of people jump right into the "I have to lose weight" mode and do all these crazy different things. It's not about losing weight. That will come. Think about fueling your body and absorbing every nutrient to help you grow stronger and more vibrant than ever.

Detox: The Good. The Bad. And the Ugly.

When we start to get healthy and commit to consuming living foods, these cells start to dump out the sludge and toxins in our system. As they are circulating through our system we are bound to have reactions also known as detox symptoms. The good thing is: as these new healthy living foods move through the body, they act like a broom and sweep out the debris.

Unfortunately, the symptoms can be uncomfortable.

In some cases, detox symptoms can include acne breakouts, a white-coated tongue, oral ulcers, a bit of hair loss, and aching joints. You can have brain fog, experience irritability, and road rage and confusion. Even the remnants of old over-the-counter drugs and prescriptions that have been embedded in the cells can make an appearance again. You can have massive headaches, blurred vision, stuffiness, and mucus. All of this is your body trying to eliminate the toxins. Let them out.

It will be over soon!

A lot of people are also wondering: How long does detox last?

In some cases, the symptoms can come in waves. You may have some today and then your body starts to calm down, but then the symptoms return a few days later. Just remember, your body is working its way back to a healthy state. It's starting to regenerate the cells on a deeper level. Just like a fish tank, you start by cleaning the water. It gets murky and cloudy and it takes a bit to clear out. The algae under the rocks and hidden in the corners of the tank will clear out if you give it time. It all really depends on how much cleansing is required to get back to a healthy, clear and clean state.

Just remember: Your health is in your own hands. When you start taking personal responsibility for what you consume, you can change your health forever and never have to go back. You have the power to heal from within!

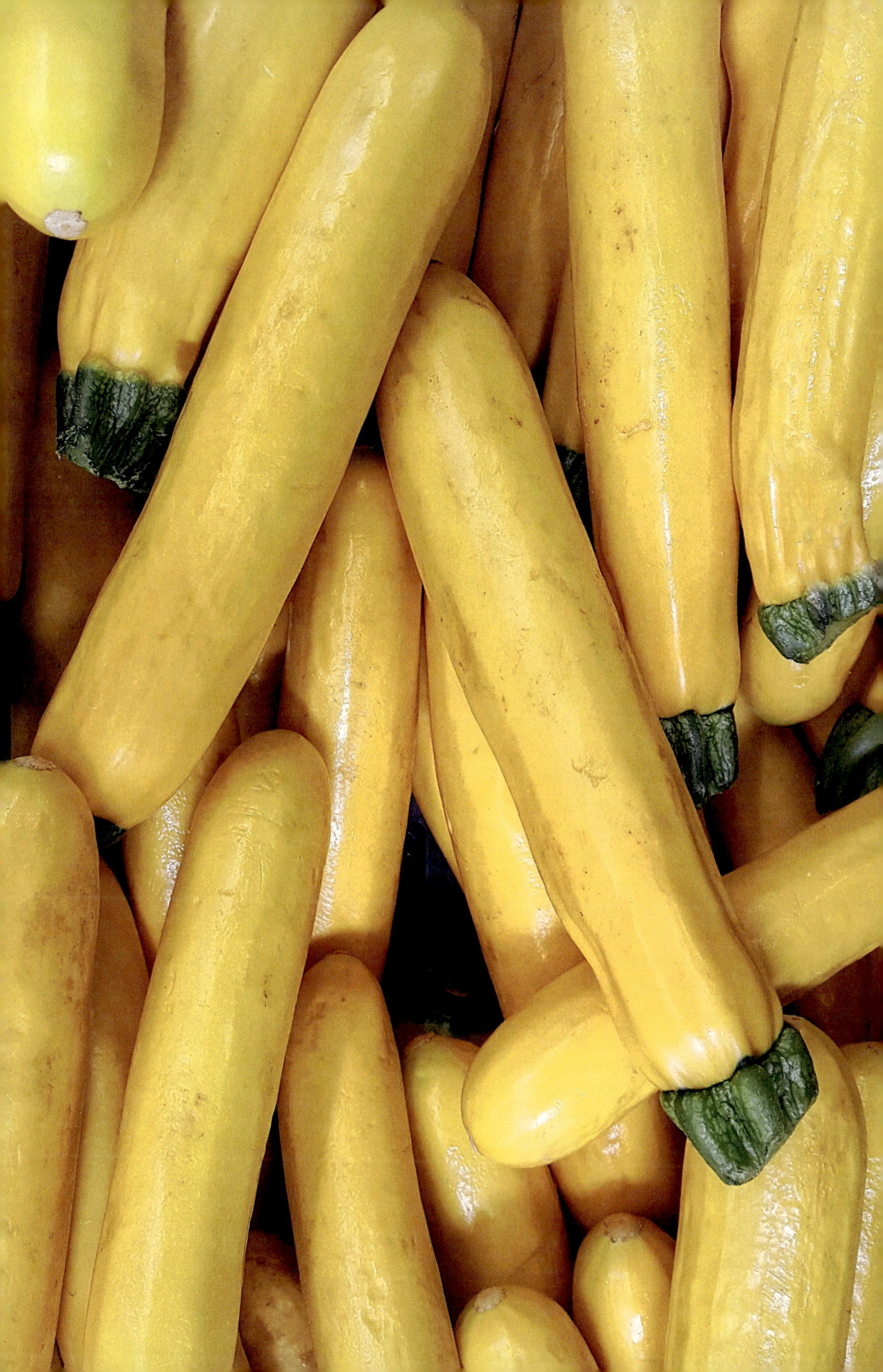

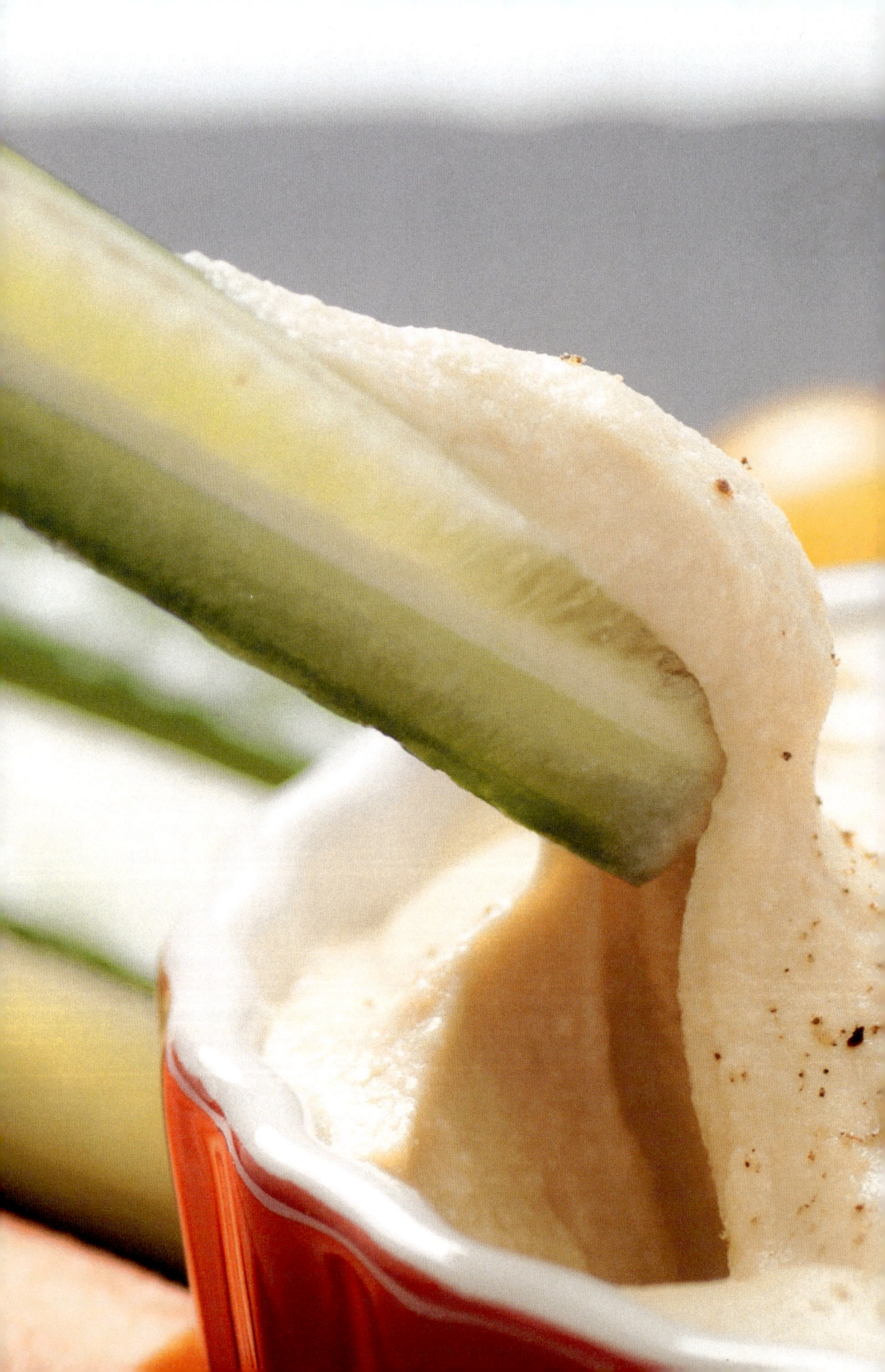

Dips, Dressings, Sauces & Soups

Crunchy, smooth, sweet, spicy, tart, savoury—any way you want it, raw vegan has it.

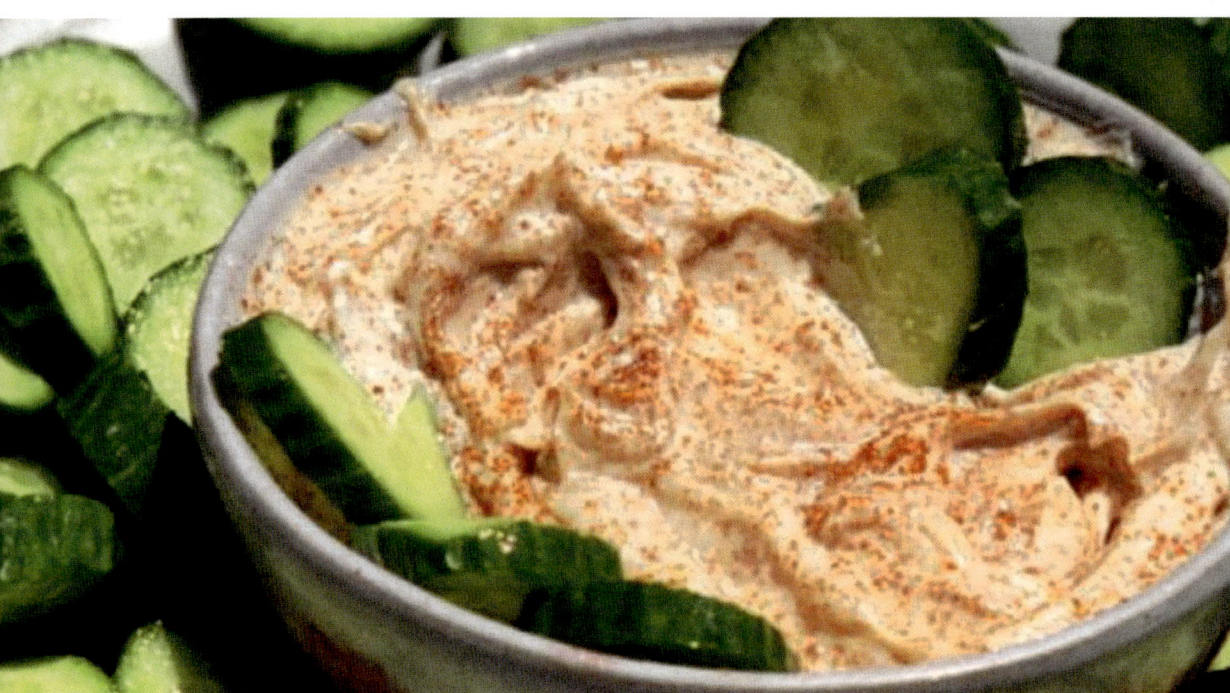

Cukes & Cream Dipping Sauce

1 c zucchini, peeled

2 TBS lemon juice

1 TBS lucuma powder

½ tsp kelp sprinkles

3 TBS raw hulled hemp hearts

Dried dill to taste

Blend with a tad bit of water. Add a dash of cayenne to taste. Scoop with cucumbers.

Nutty Nori Roll Dipping Sauce

¼ c walnuts

1 peeled lemon

1 c zucchini, peel for nice color and consistency

1 TBS wakame seaweed

1 clove of garlic

1 date (optional)

Dash of cayenne

Soak walnuts for 2 hours.

Blend in water to desired consistency.

Use fresh nori rolls for dipping. Pack them with green onions, julienned celery, sprouts, and carrots.

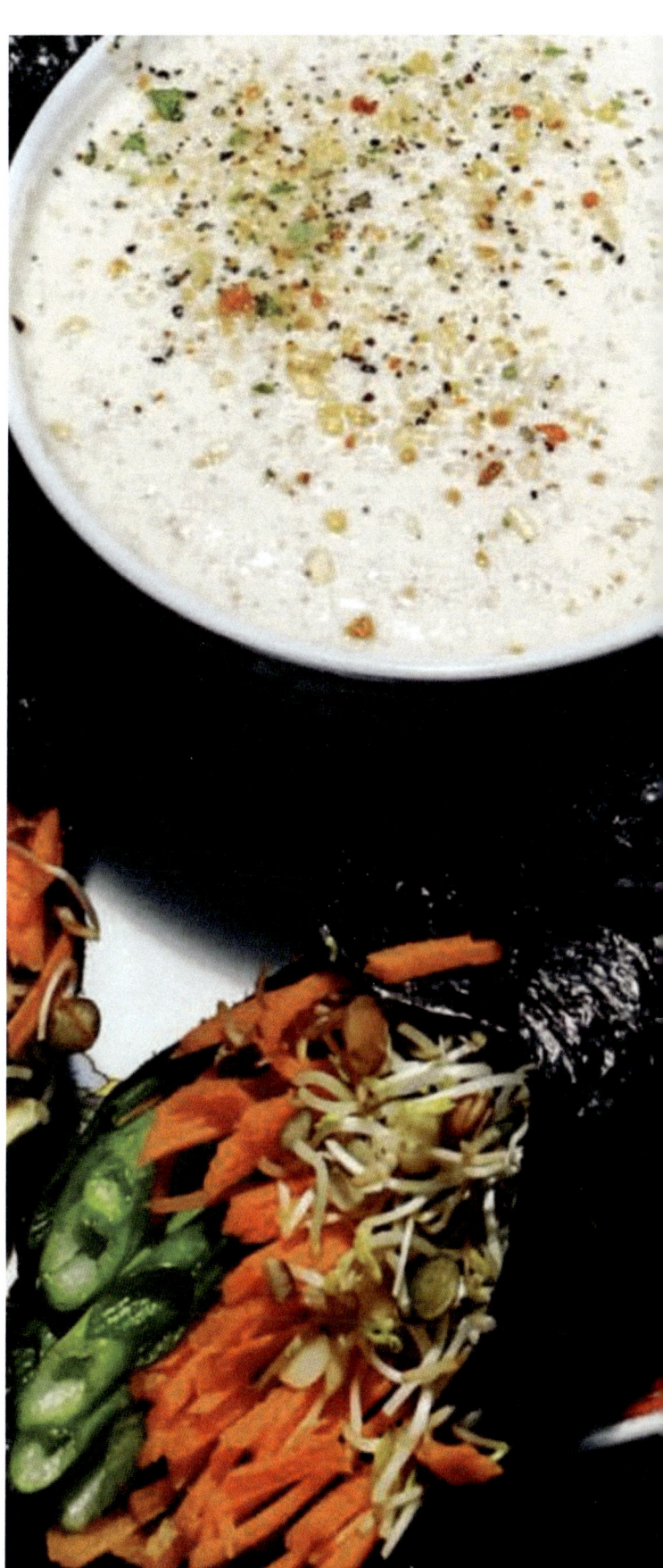

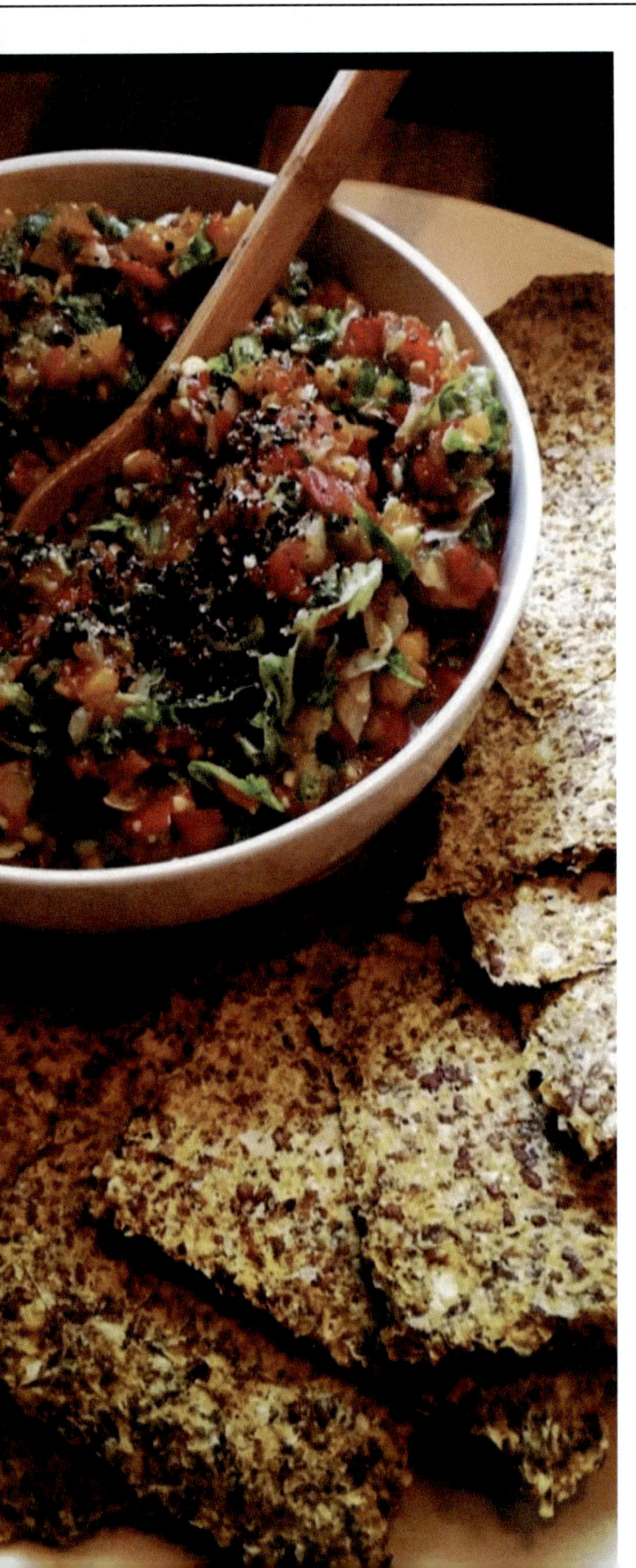

Simple Salsa

2 c tomatoes

1 c red bell peppers, chopped

½ c orange and yellow bell peppers, chopped

½ avocado, minced

2 TBS dulse leaves, chopped small

½ c finely diced Napa cabbage

Add fresh cilantro and dill to taste

Mash together well and add a dash of black cracked pepper to top.

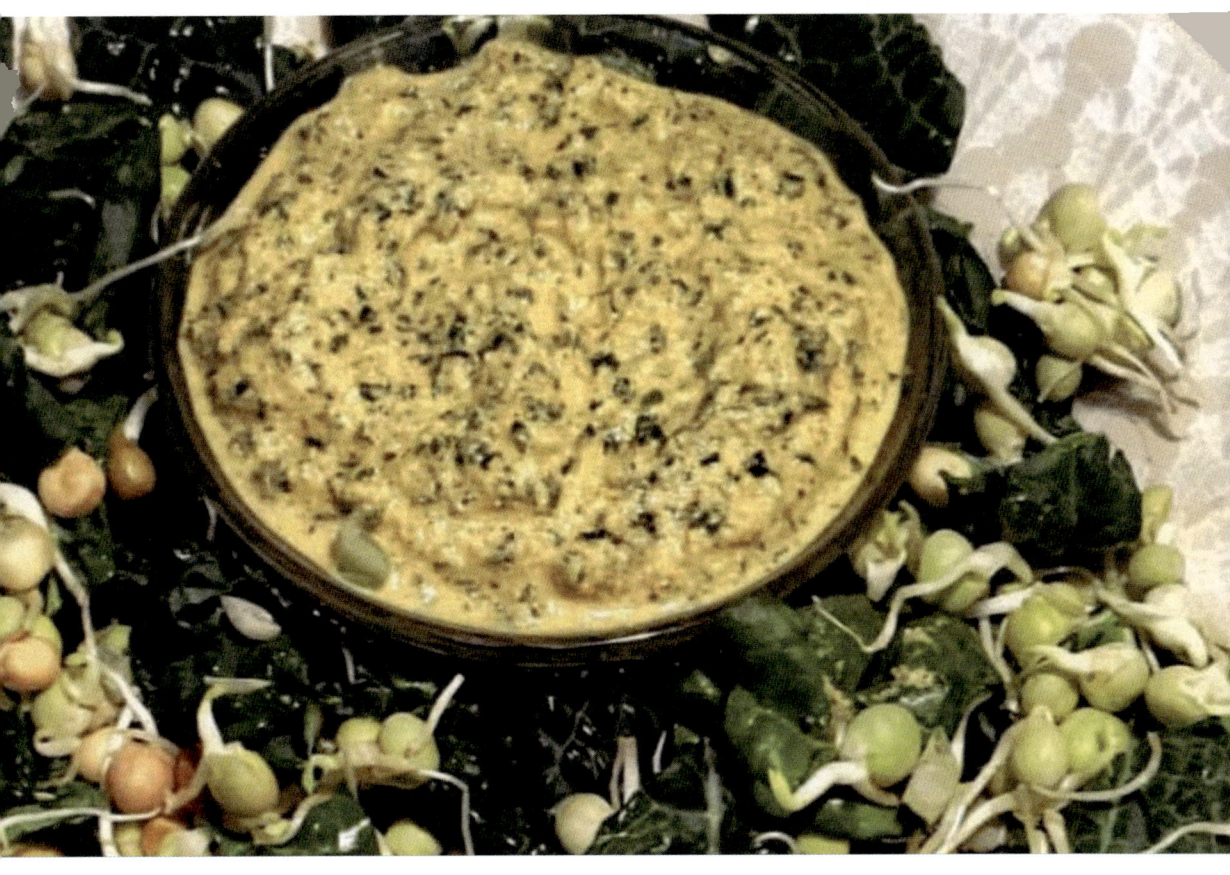

Blood-Orange Butterfly Dressing

½ c celery

½ c zucchini, peeled

1 blood orange

1 orange bell pepper

1 TBS lucuma powder (to thicken with no fat)

1 TBS Mexican Fiesta Frontier Seasoning

1 TBS wakame seaweed

Blend to smooth. Add wakame at the end and pulse.

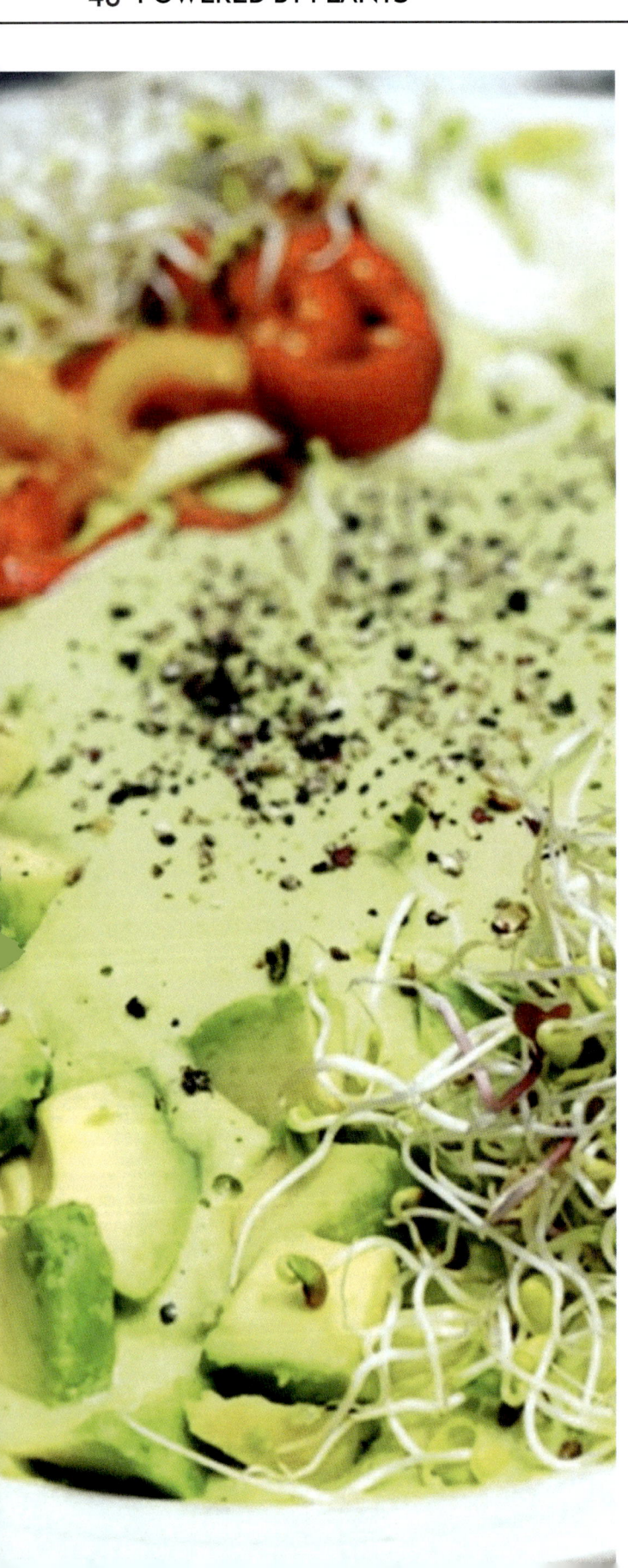

Avocado Dip

1 lemon, squeezed

½ avocado, cubed

Dulse leaves with tri-colored cracked pepper

1 c red and orange bell peppers

Blend to desired consistency.

Smooth + Savoury Tomato Dip

3 Roma tomatoes

1 red bell pepper with seeds (for spicy)

1 lemon, juiced

1 stalk of celery

½ tsp of kelp sprinkles

1 ½ TBS almond butter

Blend to smooth. Sprinkle red pepper flakes on top.

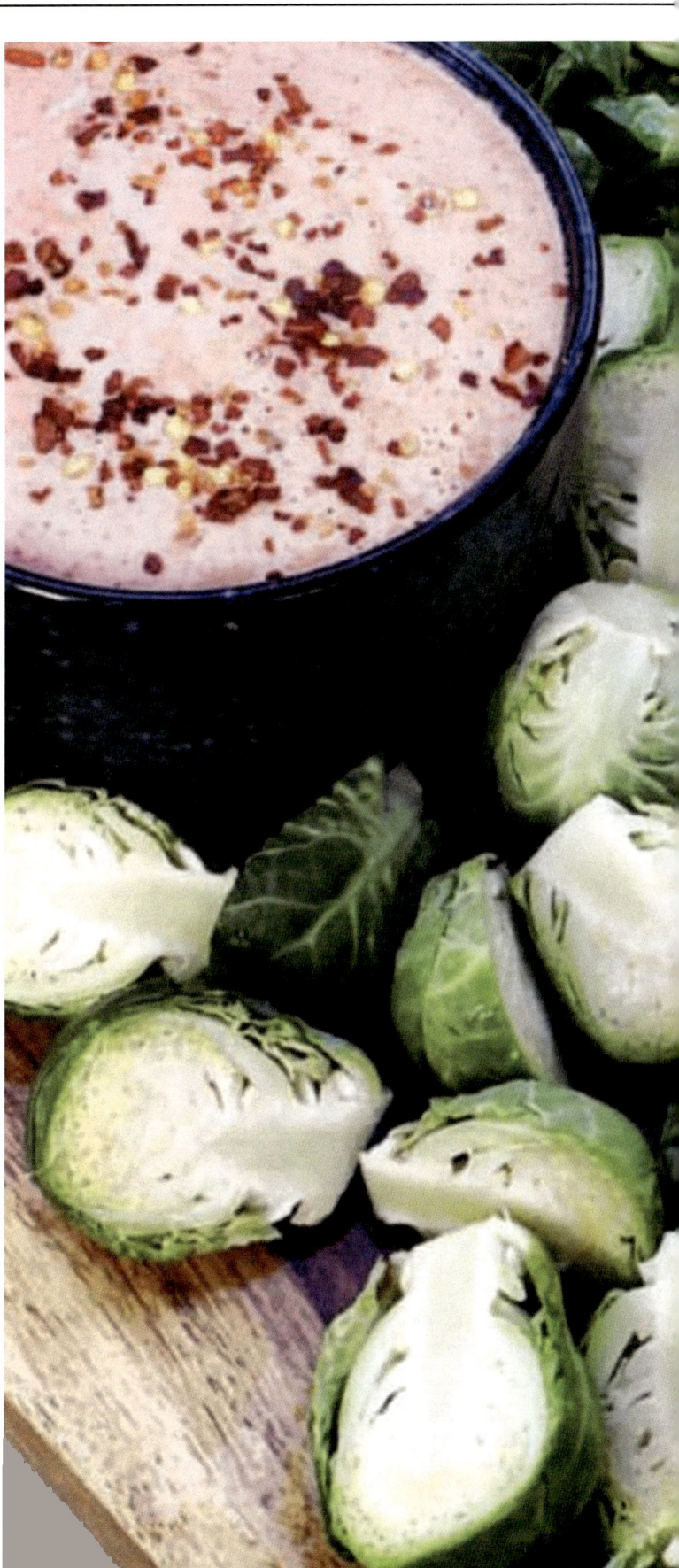

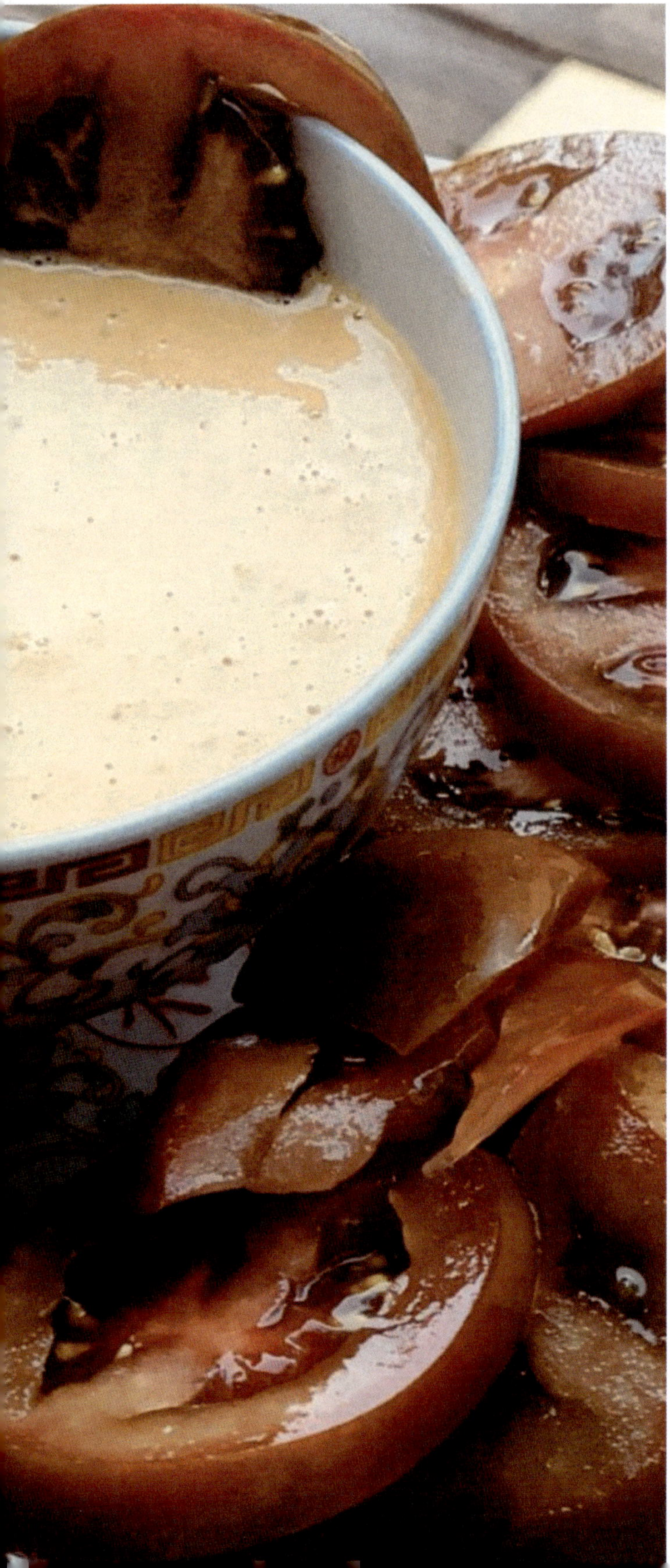

My Sweet 'N Smooth Dipping Dressing

2 ½ c bell peppers (red, yellow, orange), chopped

1 lemon, squeezed

1 ½ TBS tahini

1 TBS dulse flakes

Dash of Frontier Garlic and Herb Blend Seasoning

Blend with water to desired consistency.

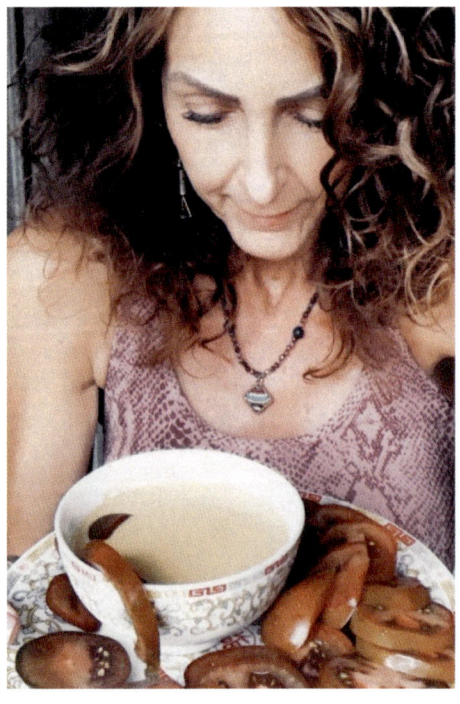

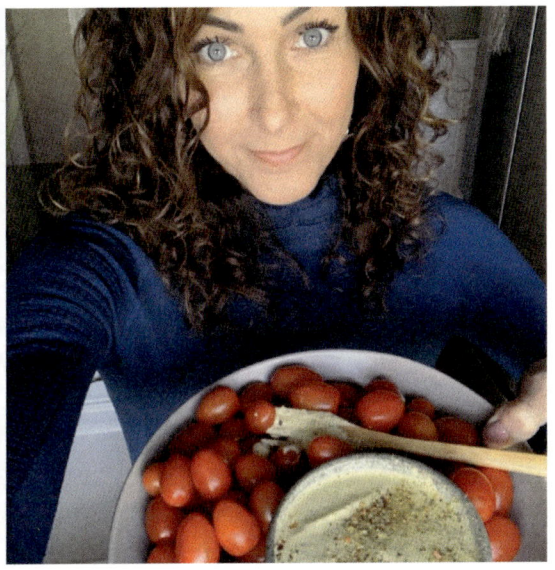

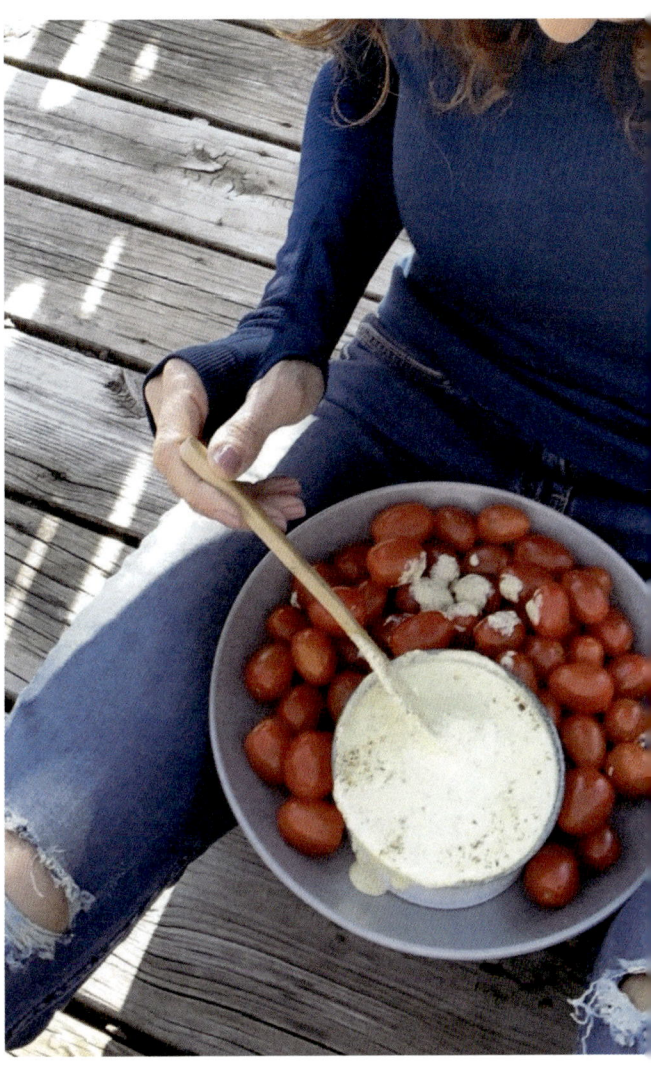

Yummy Yellow Squash Dip

1 c yellow squash, peeled

1 TBS tahini

2 TBS raw hulled hemp-seed hearts

½ tsp kelp granulars

3 dried apricots, unsulphured

One clove of garlic, minced (optional)

Blend well and add water to taste.

Add cayenne pepper to taste.

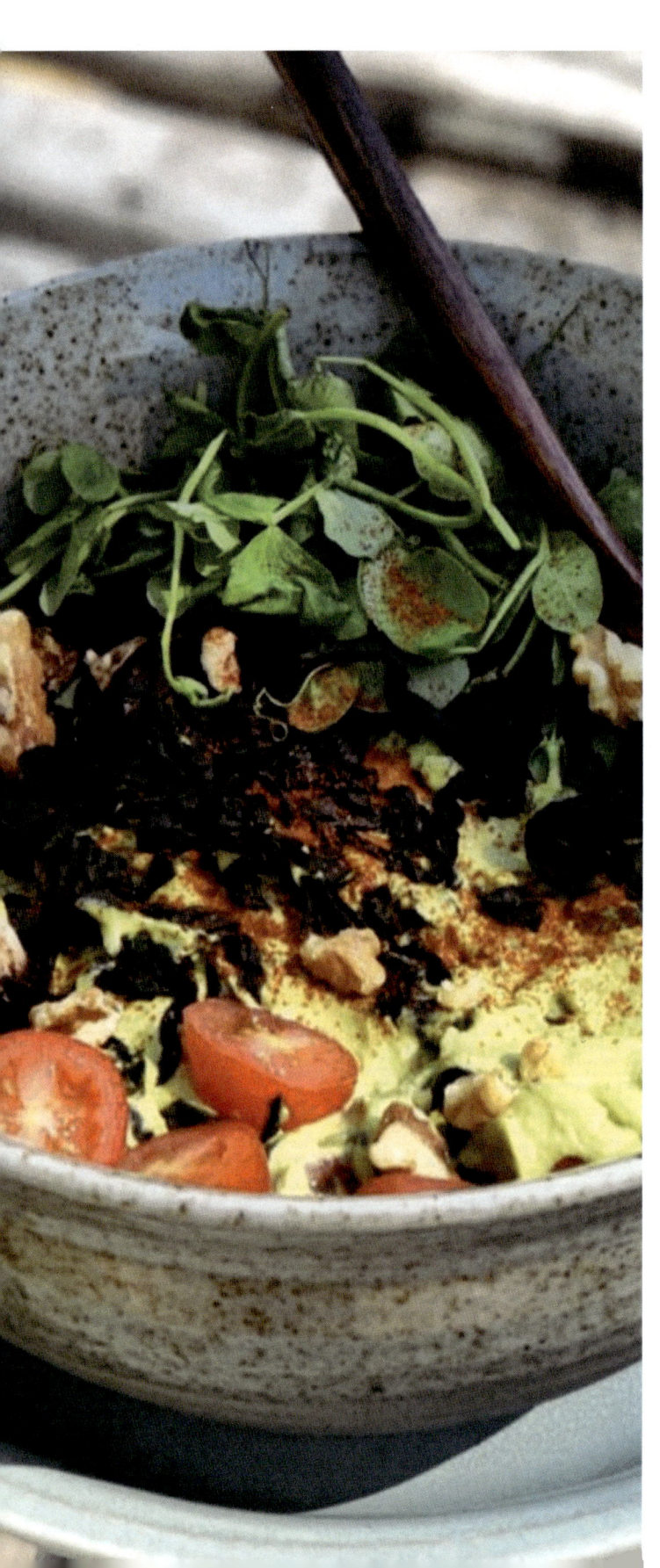

Easy Peasy Dip

1 ½ lbs raw peas, soaked for one hour in warm water

¼ c raw walnuts, soaked for two hours

1 lemon, juiced

Dash of cayenne to taste

1 TBS Frontier Garlic and Herb Seasoning

1 TBS wakame seaweed, rinsed

Blend in a high-speed blender to smooth consistency. Gently warm the soup in the blender to no more than 115 degrees Fahrenheit.

Hearty Carrot Soup

1 large tomato

1 lemon, peeled

2—3 inches hot banana pepper to taste

2 c chopped carrots

2 c celery

1 tsp garlic powder

½ TBS smoked paprika

1-inch fresh ginger

½ avocado

Blend all in a high-speed blender except the avocado.

Blend warm to touch but still raw under 115 degrees Fahrenheit.

After everything is blended to smooth pulse, gently blend the avocado in. Top with little crunchy veggies like diced okra.

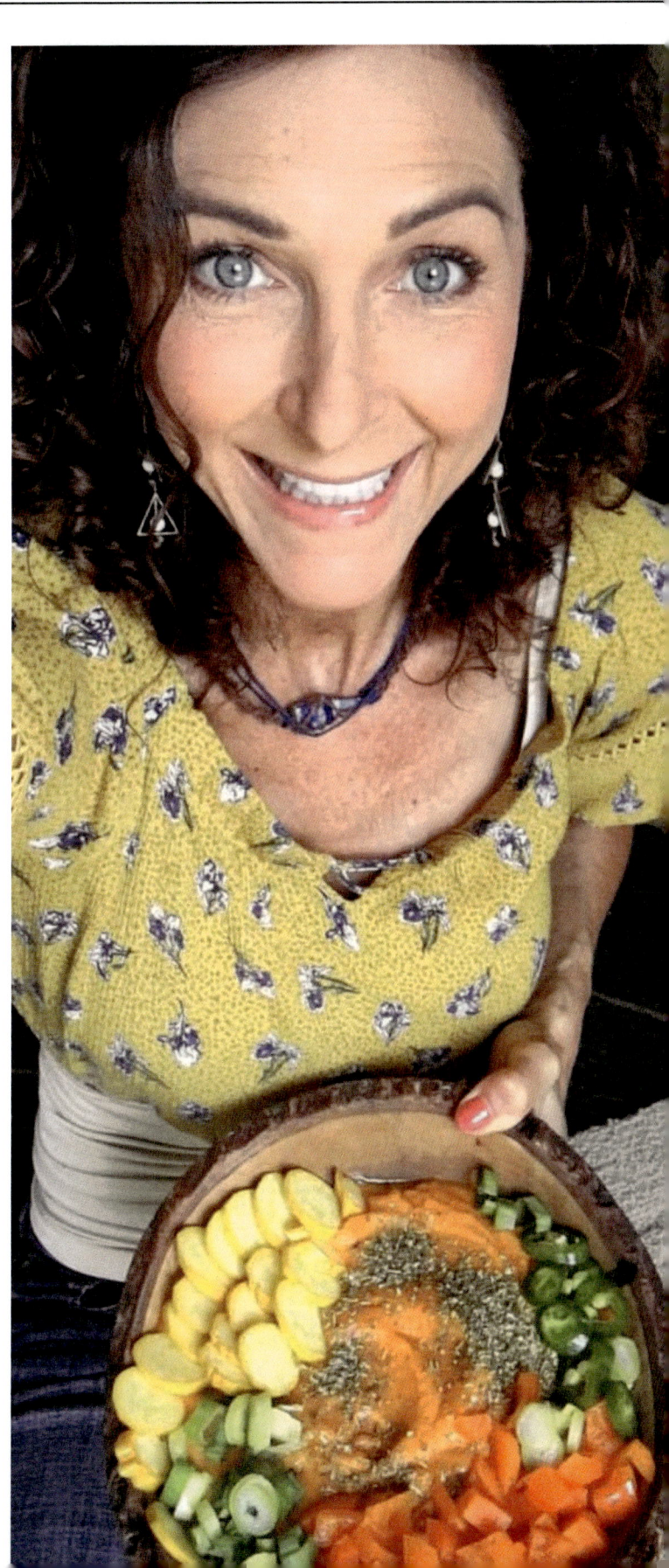

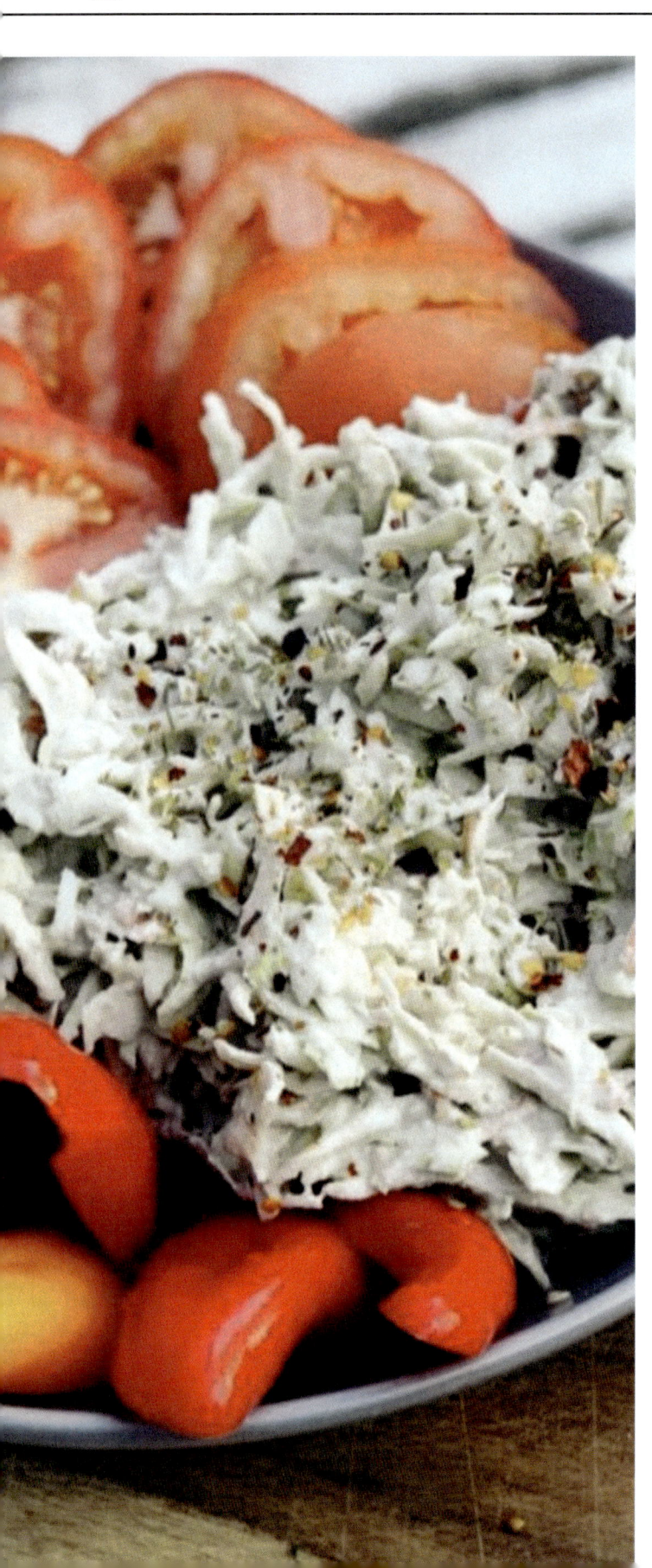

Simple Slaw

Base:

5 c green or purple Napa cabbage, diced or grated

Sauce:

1 zucchini, peeled

½ c celery

¼ c almonds or walnuts

1 TBS wakame seaweed or a dash of himalayan salt

3 TBS apple cider vinegar

1 TBS lemon juice or 1 TBS dill

Dash of red pepper flakes and tri-colored ground peppercorn

Soak the almonds or walnuts in warm water for two hours. Drain.

Add a bit of water and blend at high speed for best results.

Combine with cabbage.

Savoury Slaw

1 c carrots

1 c cherry tomatoes

1 TBS wakame seaweed

3 TBS lemon juice

1 TBS tahini

2 TBS raw hulled hemp hearts

Cayenne to taste

Combine with cabbage and sprouts.

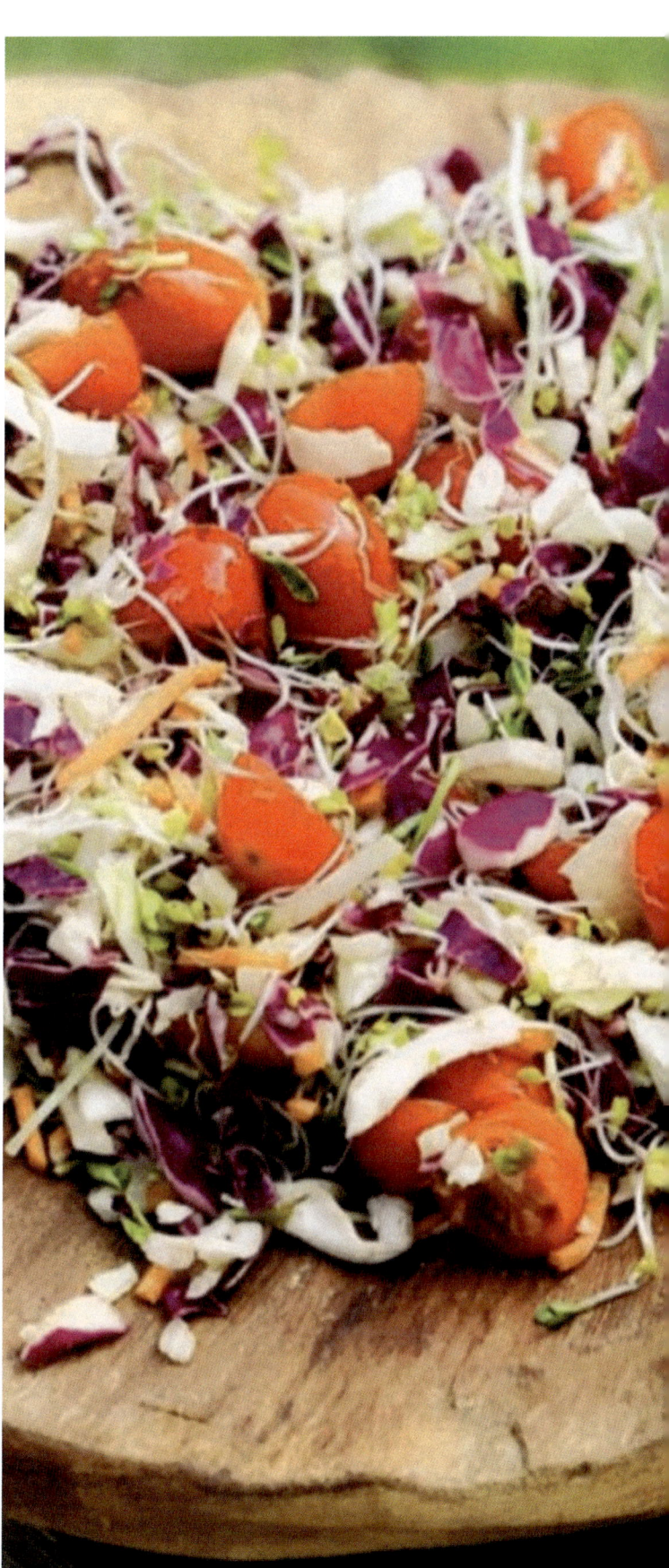

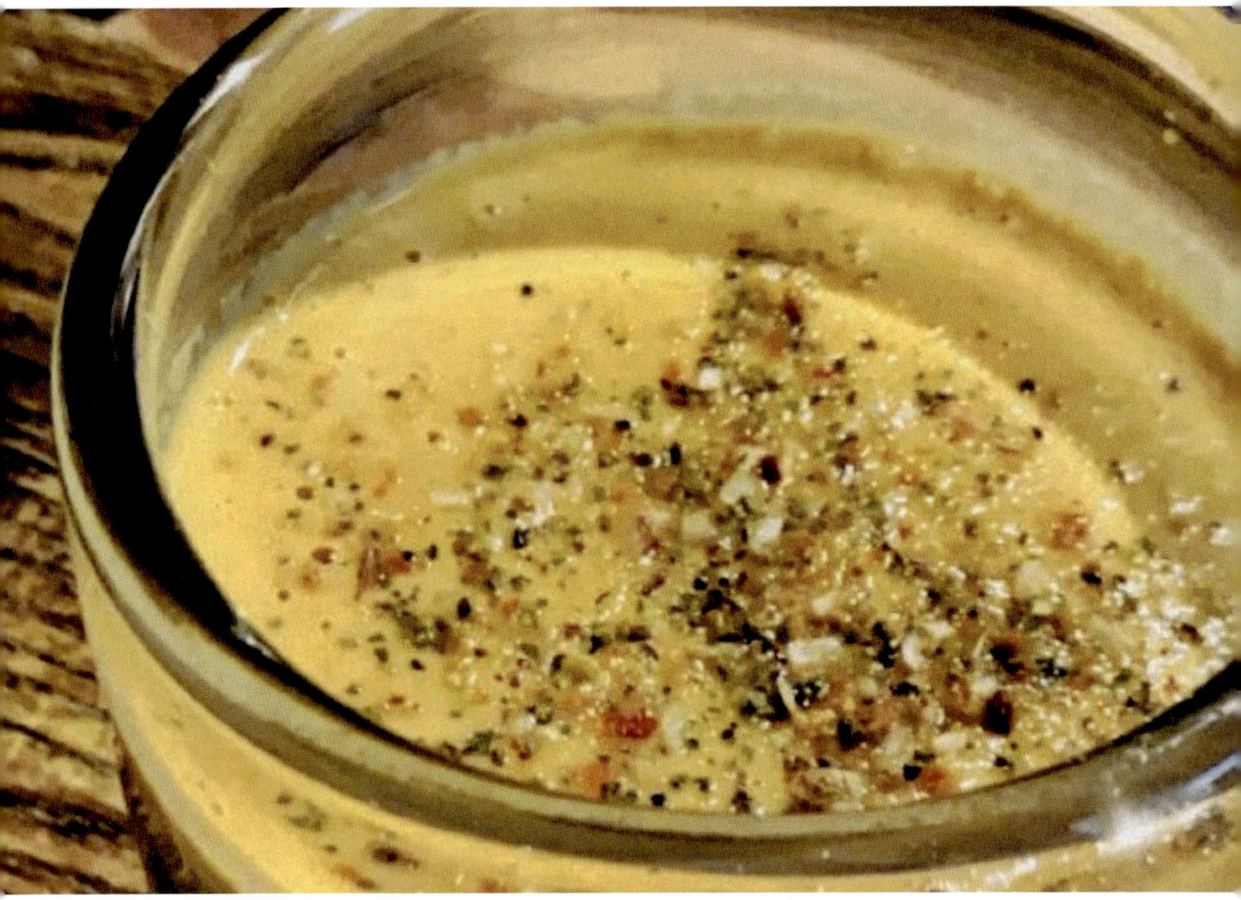

Tanny's So-Simple Sauce

2 ½ c bell peppers (red, yellow and orange), chopped

1 lemon, squeezed

1 ½ TBS almond butter

1 TBS dulse flakes

Dash of Frontier Garlic and Herbs Blend Seasoning

Water to thin if needed.

Blend to smooth.

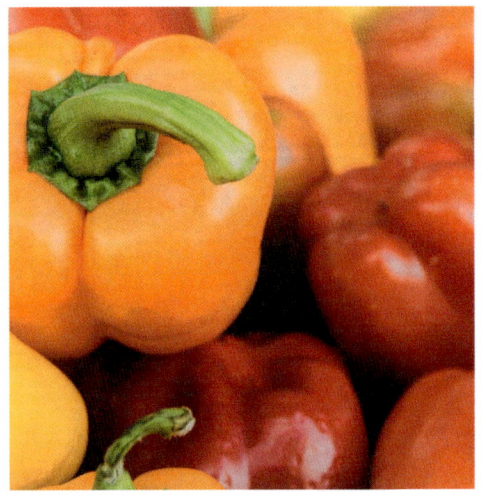

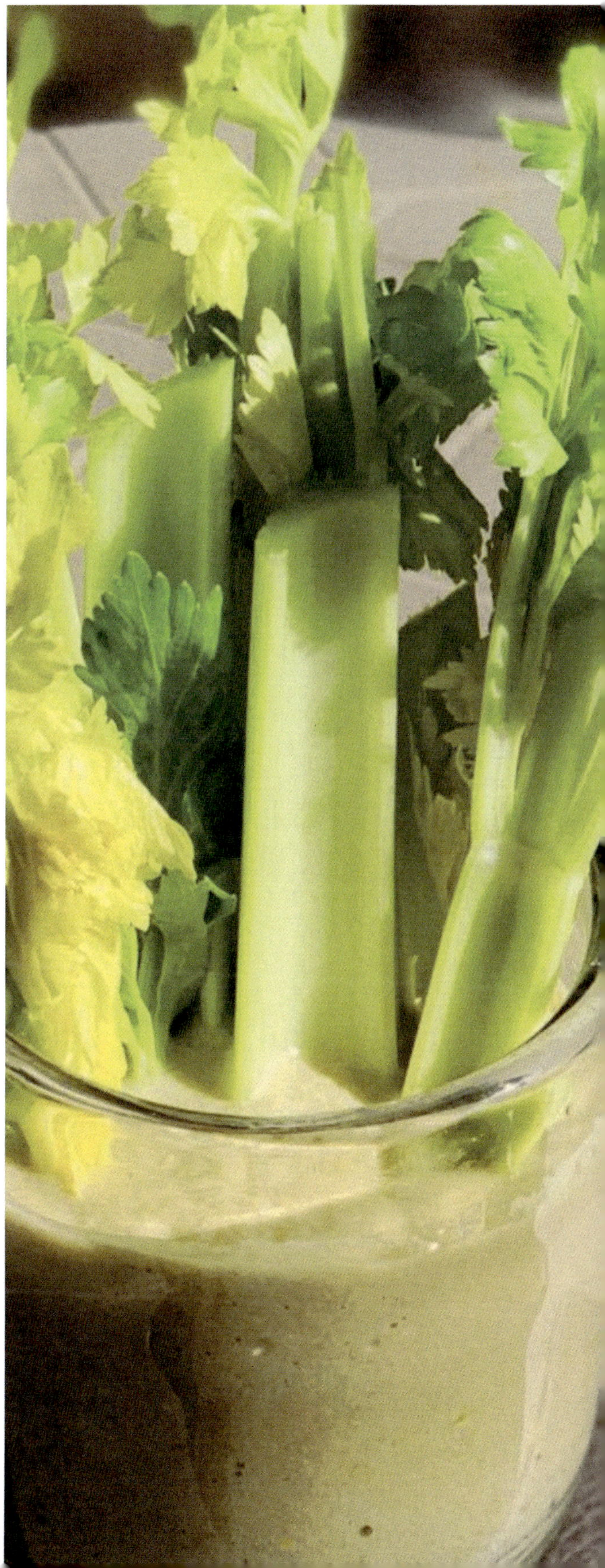

Tahini Treat Dipping Sauce

1 c zucchini, peeled

1 TBS tahini

1 lemon, juiced

2 dates, pitted

1 TBS dulse flakes

1 clove of garlic

Add water and blend to desired consistency.

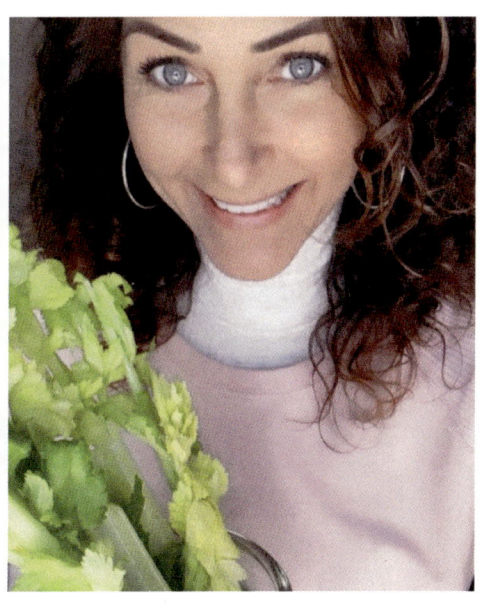

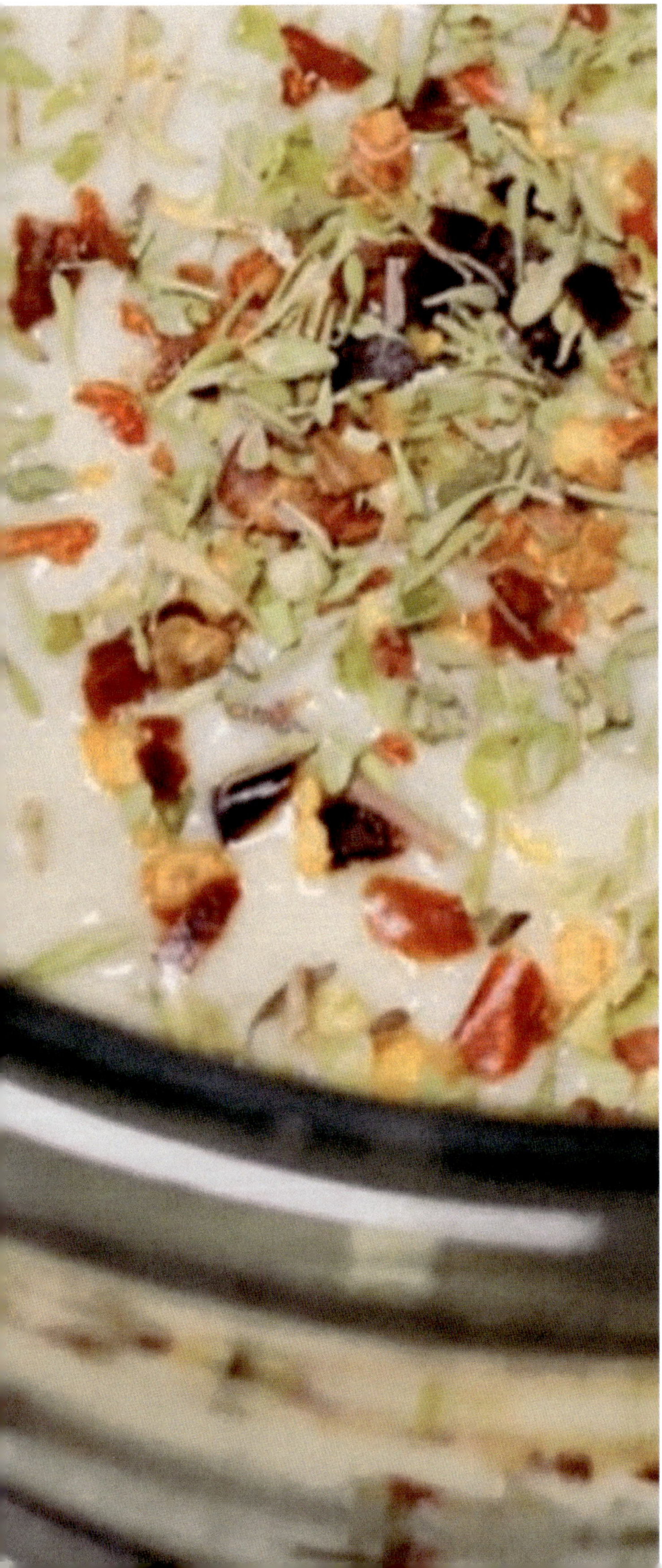

Creamy Pumpkin Seed Dressing

1 c celery, light part

½ c zucchini, peeled

¼ c raw pumpkin seeds, soaked for 1 hour

1 lemon, squeezed

1 TBS dulse flakes

Dash of Frontier Garlic and Herb Blend Seasoning

Blend with water to thin.

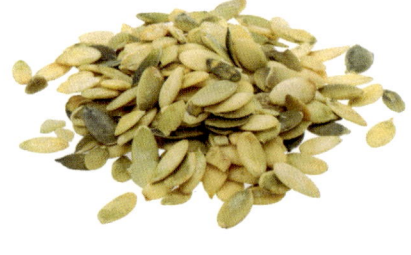

Sweet & Zesty Dipping Sauce/ Dressing

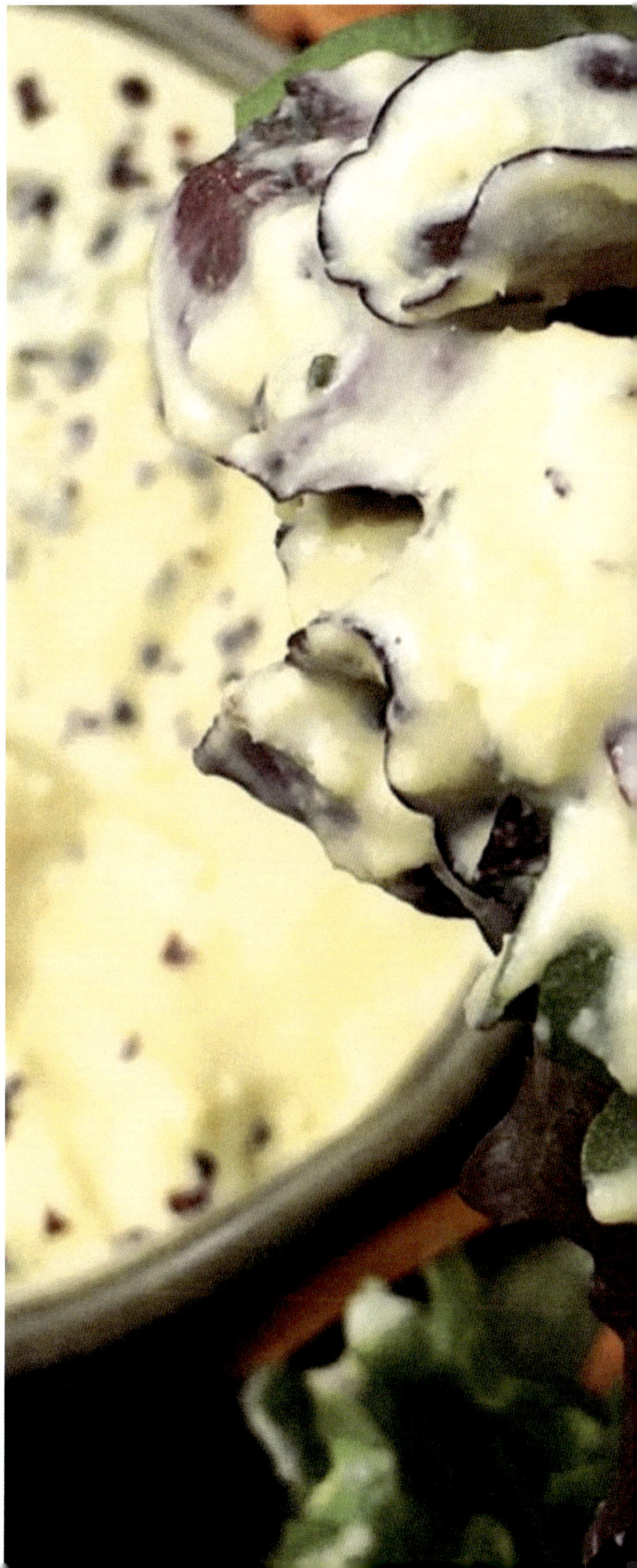

1 c yellow peppers, chopped

1 c celery (light part), chopped

½ lemon, peeled

1 date, pitted

1 TBS lucuma powder

3 TBS raw hulled hemp-seed hearts

1 TBS dulse flakes, pulsed at the end

Blend with water to desired consistency.

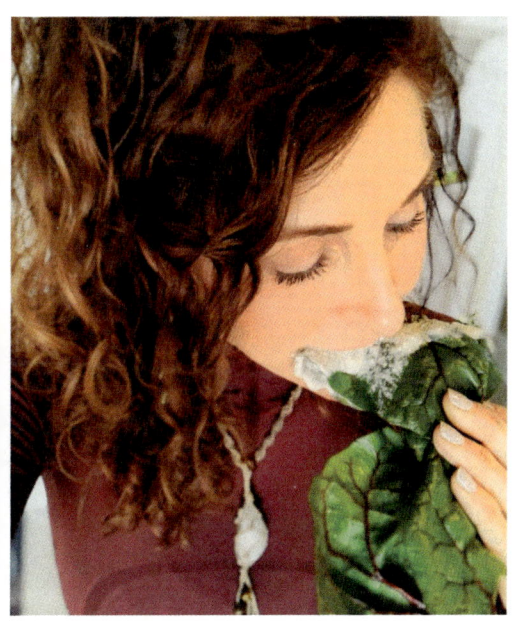

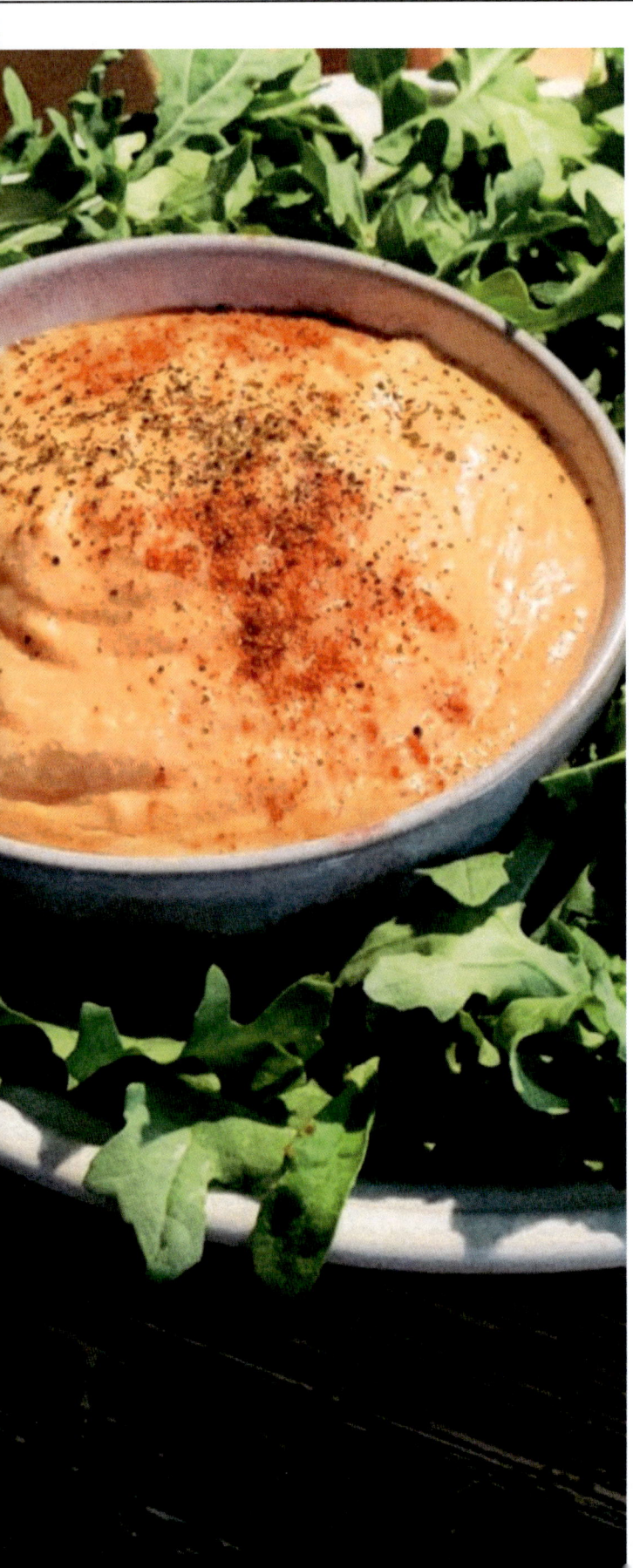

On A Coconut Kick

¼ c raw coconut

2 dates

1 yellow bell pepper

¾ c Roma tomatoes

2 TBS lemon juice

½ tsp kelp sprinkles

Dash of cayenne

Add water and blend to desired consistency.

Hemp Seed Heart Salad Dressing

2 TBS raw hulled hemp seed hearts

1 c carrots

1 c cherry tomatoes

1 TBS wakame seaweed

3 TBS lemon juice

1 TBS tahini

Cayenne to taste

Blend to a dip or add a bit of water for a thinner dressing.

Most of my dressings have an acidic component which means they will easily last up to 4—5 days.

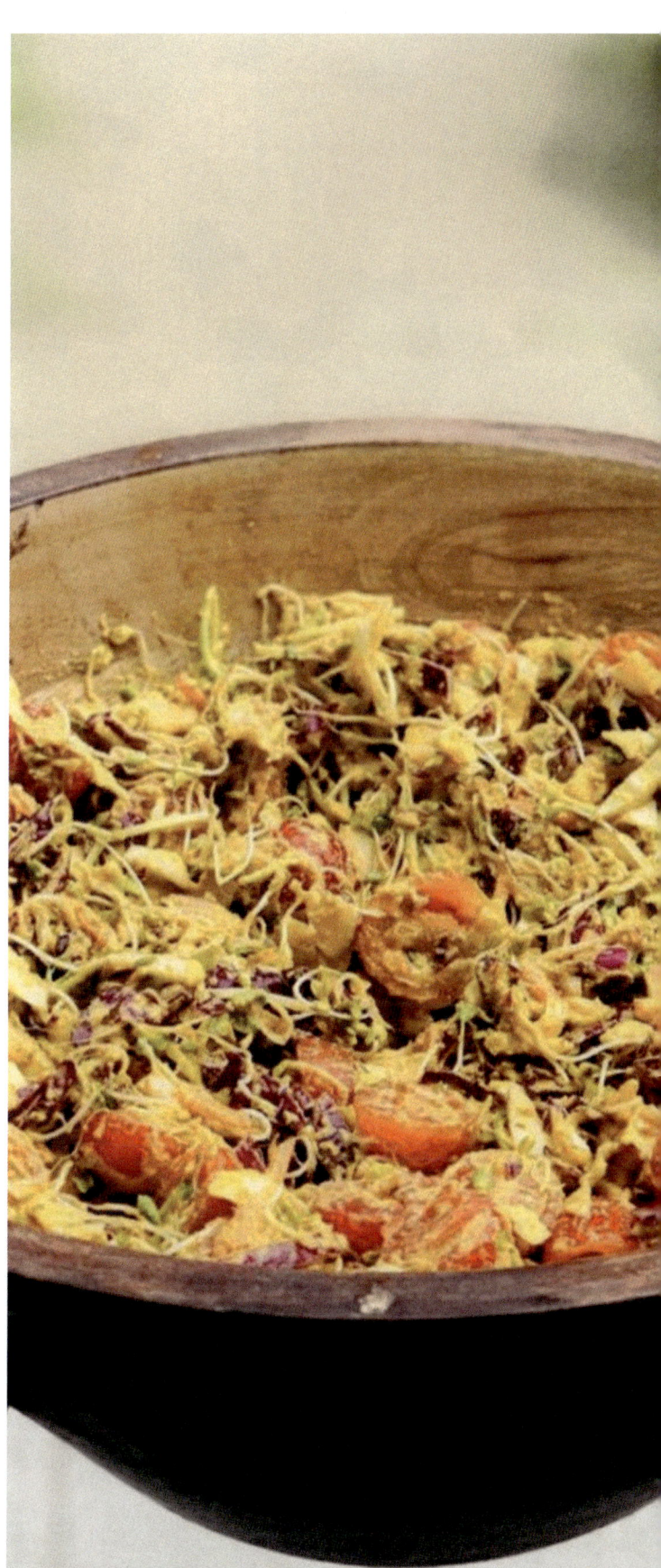

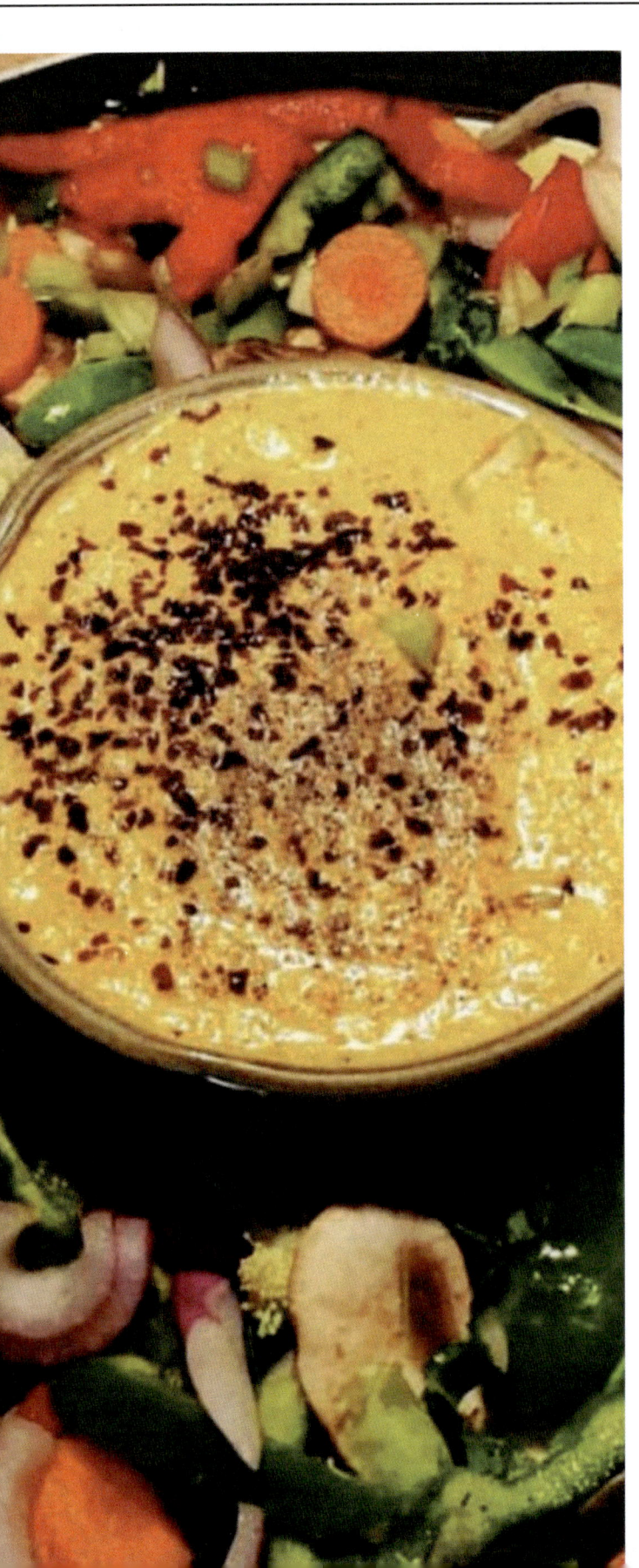

Sweet & Spicy Carrot Almond Dressing

1 c carrots

1 TBS lucuma powder

¼ c raw almonds, soaked and drained

2 TBS apple cider vinegar or lemon juice

½ TBS dulse flakes

Red pepper flakes to taste

Soak raw almonds for 8 hours. Add a tad bit of water and blend well. Season with black pepper and sprinkle dulse flakes on top.

Soften the veggies (sorted of wilted) for 30 minutes in shallow water in dehydrator at 112 degrees Fahrenheit.

Raw Vegan Sauce With A Kick

3 TBS raw hulled hemp seed hearts

¾ c zucchini, peeled

1 date, pitted

1 large lemon, juiced

⅓ TBS kelp granules

Add water to achieve desired thinness and blend well.

Season with 1/2 TBS Frontier Brand Italian Spices.

This is a great base recipe for adding in different herbs and spices to change up the flavor.

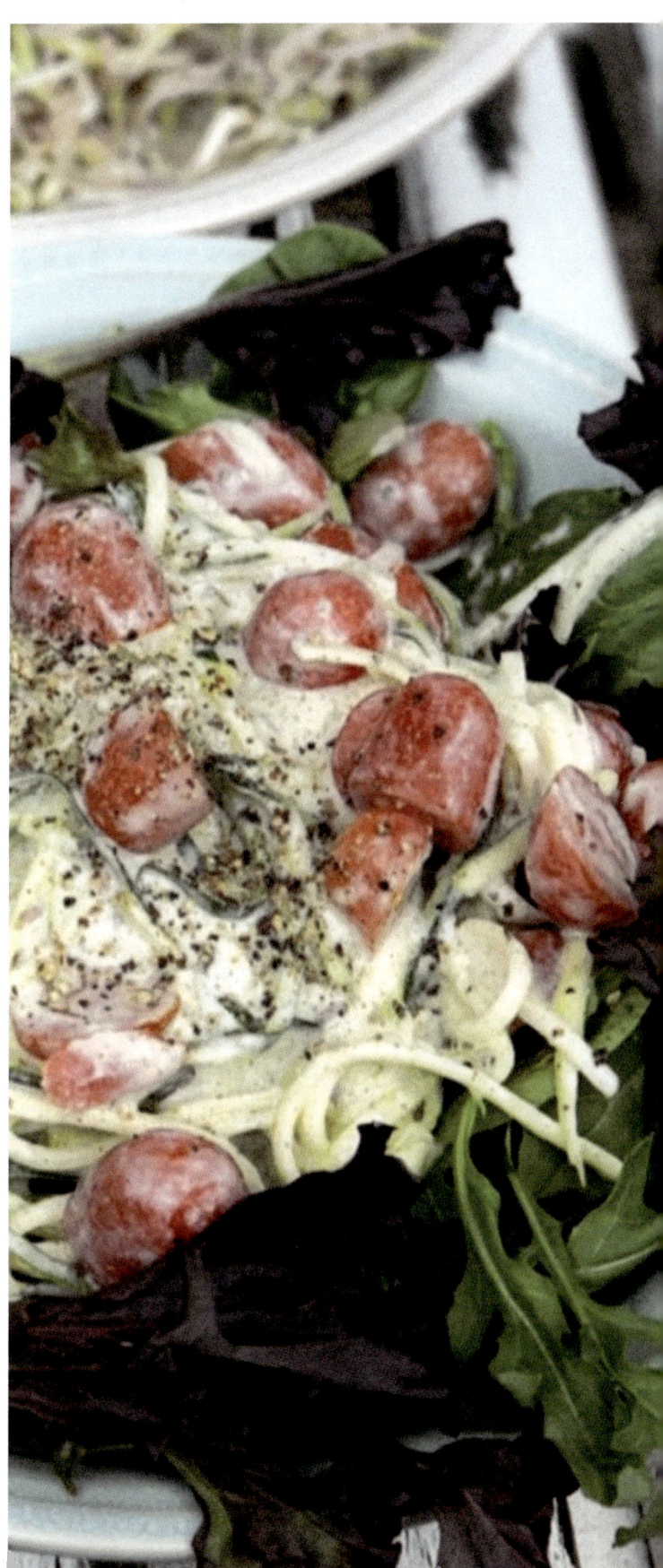

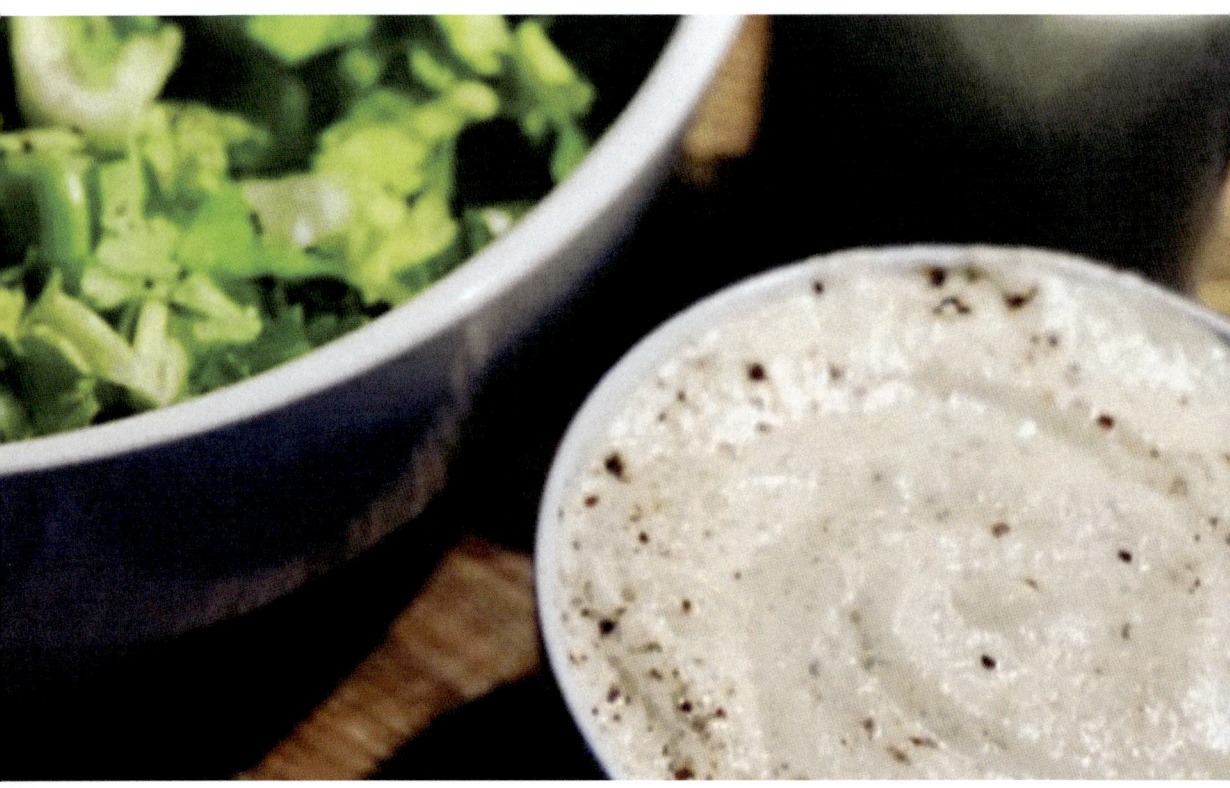

Sweet Almond Dipping Sauce

¼ c raw almonds, soaked and drained

1 lemon, squeezed

2 TBS raisins

1 c yellow squash or zucchini, peeled

⅓ tsp kelp granules

Soak almonds for 8 hours and drain. Add water and blend to desired consistency.

Stir in black pepper.

Mexican Fiesta Dip

¾ c carrots

1 c tomatoes

2 TBS tahini

1 TBS dulse flakes

½ TBS Frontier Mexican Fiesta Seasoning

Add water to achieve desired thinness and blend well.

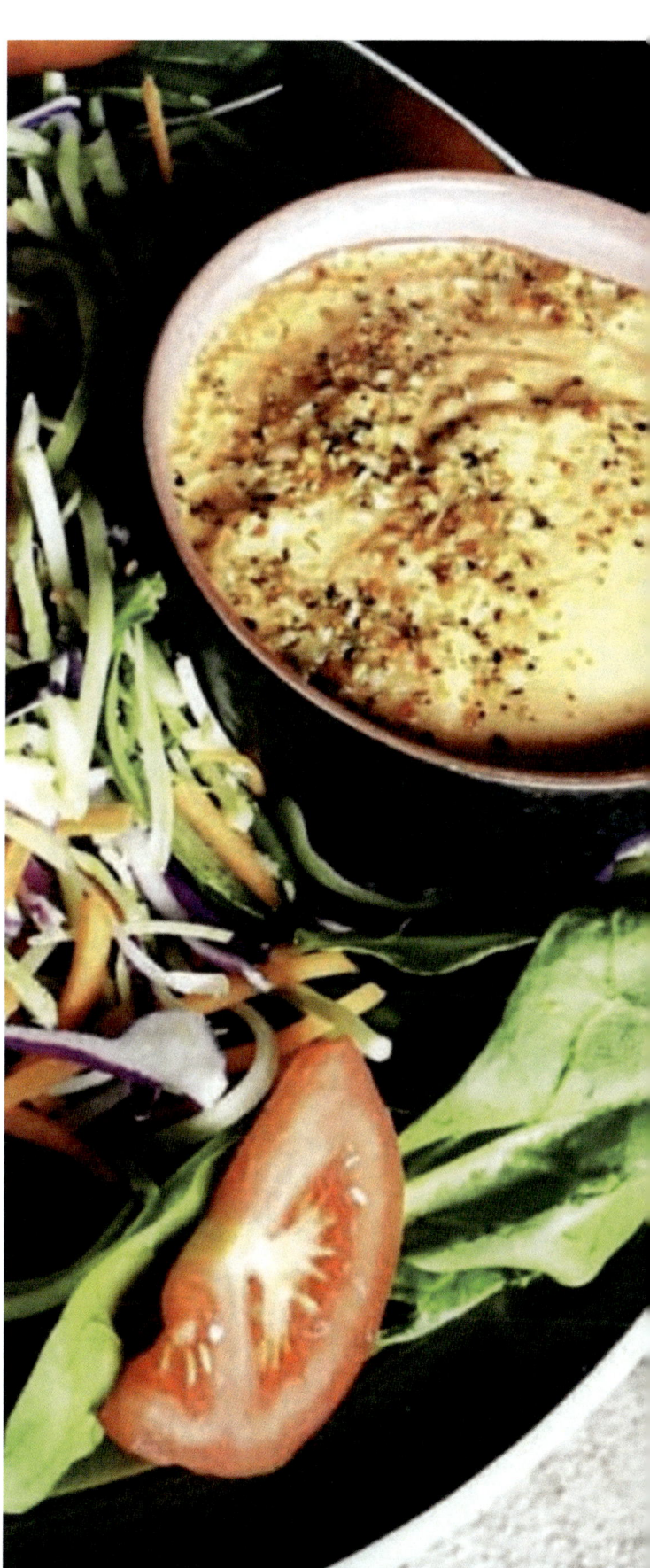

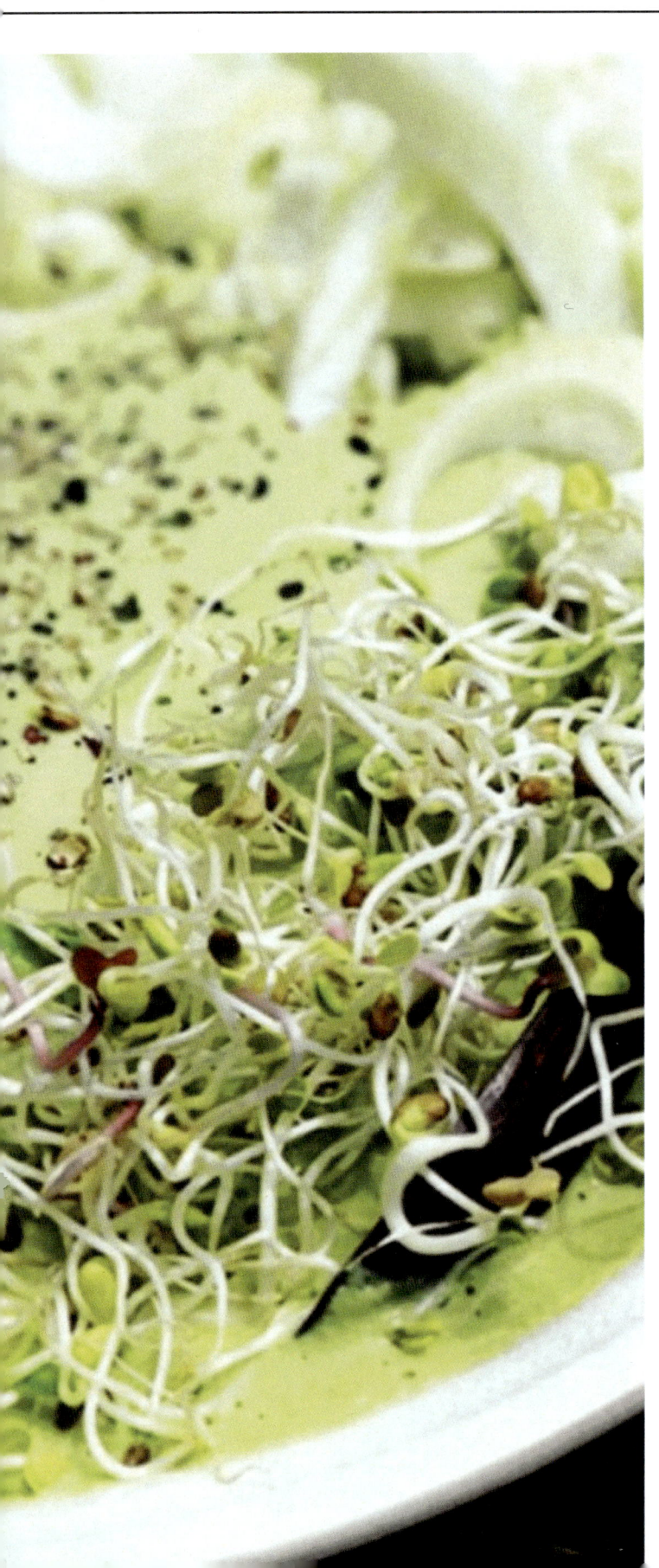

TannyRaw Fennel Pea Soup

4 c raw peas

1 c fennel bulb, diced

1 lemon, juiced

½ c celery

1 tsp kelp flakes

1 date

½ c yellow bell pepper

2 TBS tahini

Soak peas for an hour in warm water and drain. Add water to achieve desired thinness and blend to smooth a consistency.

Top with tri-color cracked pepper, sprouts, avocado, or any veggies you want!

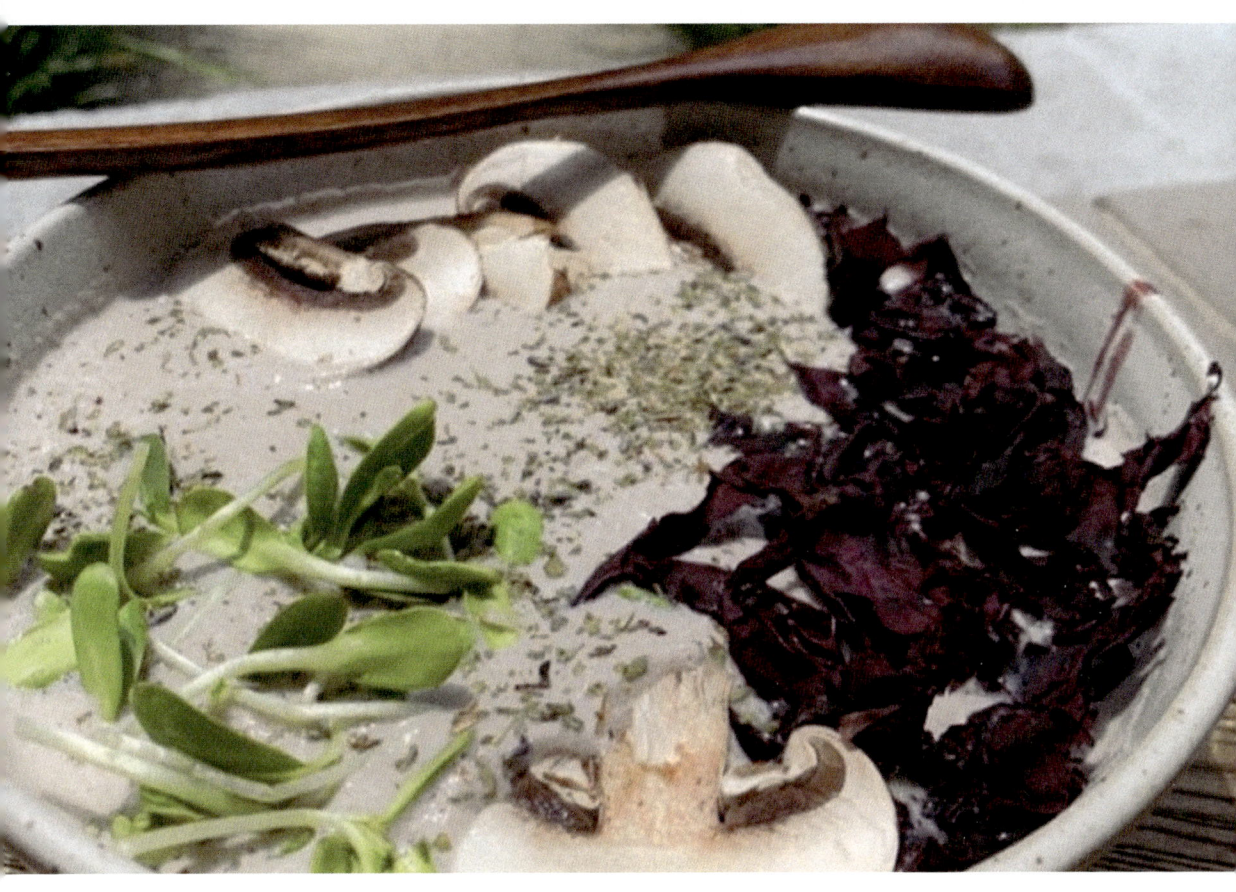

Walnut Mushroom Soup

1 c water (more for sauce)

¾ c walnuts, soaked and drained

1 c baby bella mushrooms

1 lemon, juiced

1 TBS dulse flakes or wakame seaweed

Dill to taste

1 TBS lucuma powder (optional to thicken)

2 dates

1 stick of celery (optional)

Soak almonds for 2 hours.

Blend to a smooth and creamy consistency.

Pulse in dulse or wakame seaweed.

Garnish with dried Italian seasoning, mushrooms, sunflower greens, and dulse flakes.

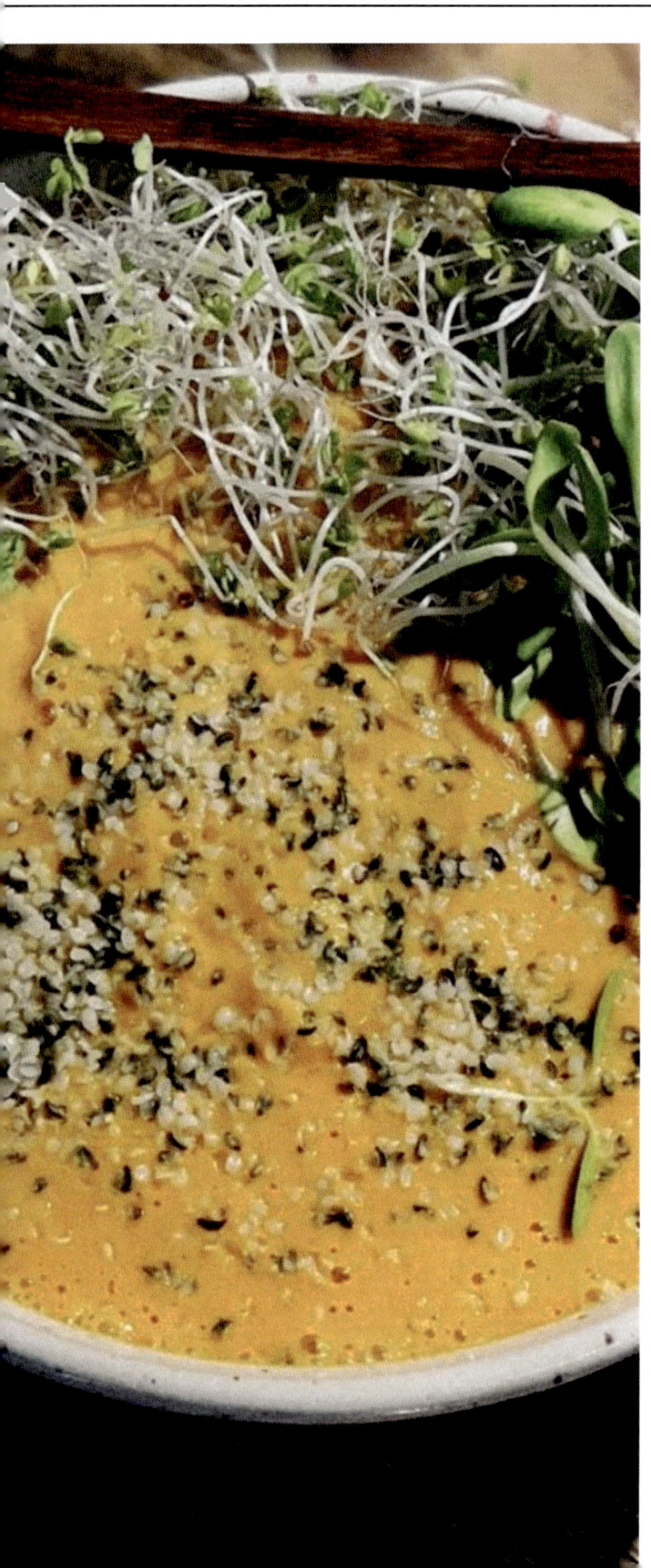

Sweet Sunshine Carrot & Tomato Soup

16 oz carrots

¾ c water

1 lemon, juiced

2 TBS dulse flakes

¼ c cherry tomatoes (optional)

2 TBS raw tahini (or other nutter butter, nuts, or seeds)

1 clove of garlic (optional)

Blend to smooth consistency. Make it warm to touch—no more than 115 degrees Fahrenheit.

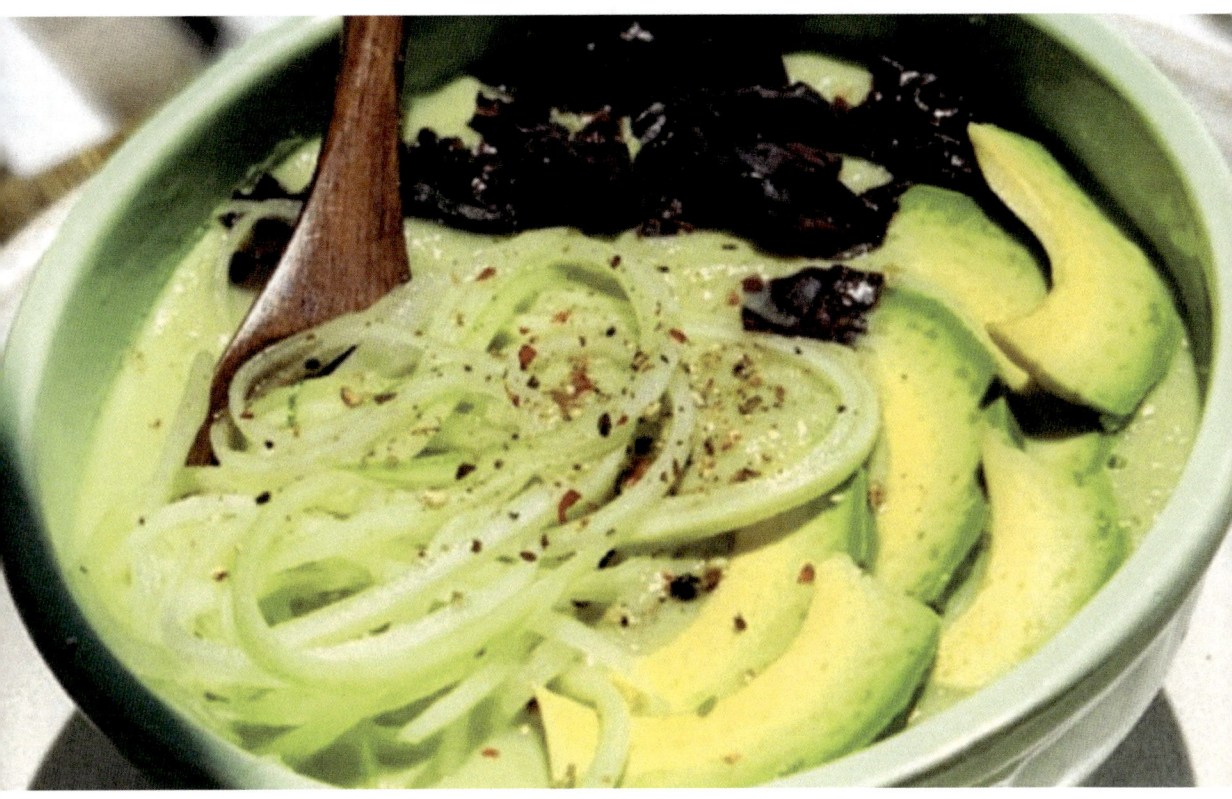

Cucumber Avocado Soup

2 c cucumber, peeled

1 c celery

2 dates

1 garlic clove

1 TBS No Salt Herb Spice by Frontier Seasonings

1 lemon, juiced

1 TBS wakame seaweed

Blend until smooth. Add water; Start with 1/2 cup and add more depending on how thin you want it.

After blended, add 1/2 avocado and blend on low just till smooth. This helps the soup remain creamy.

Note: Too much blending of the avocado creates a mousse-like texture.

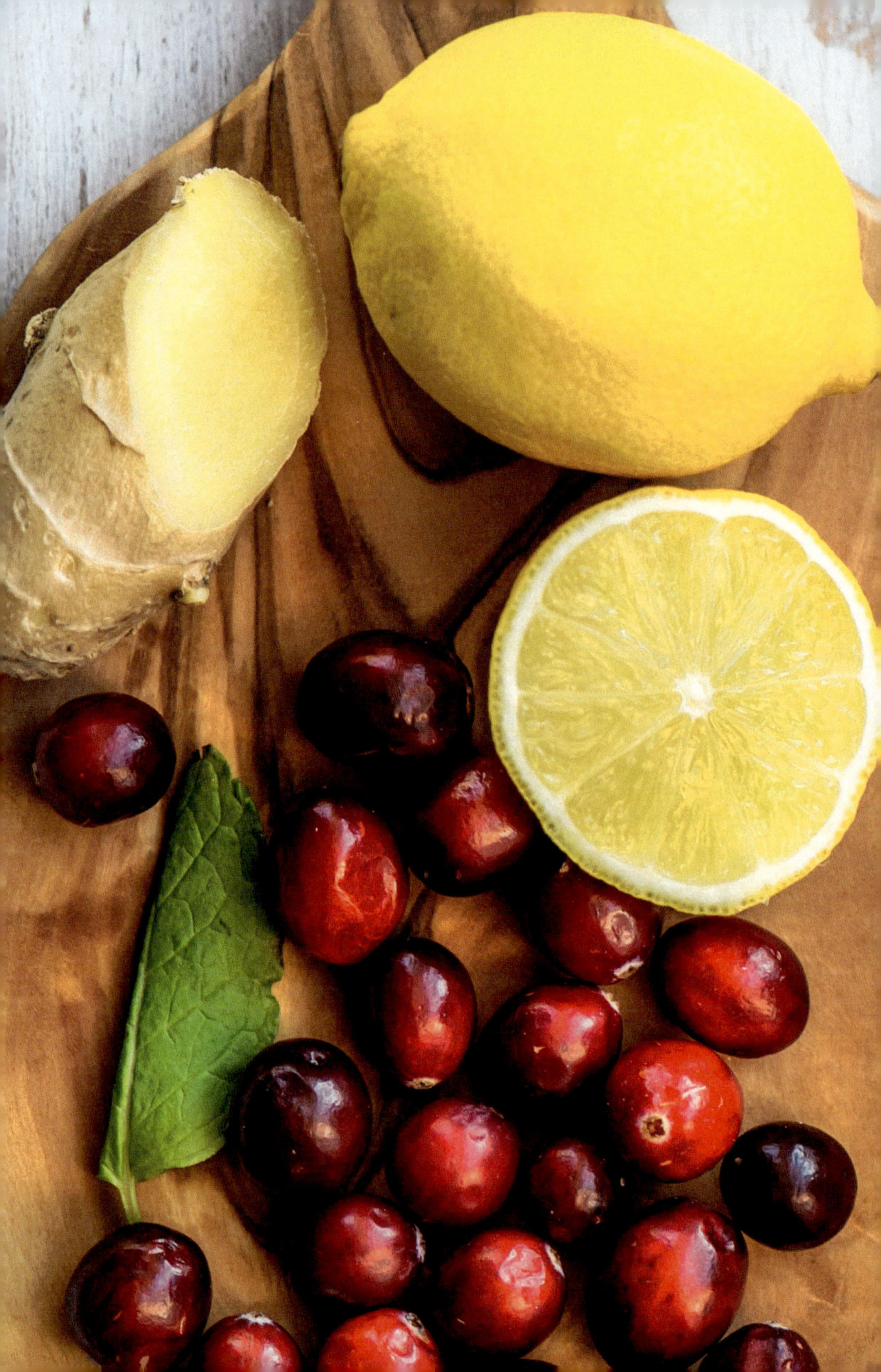

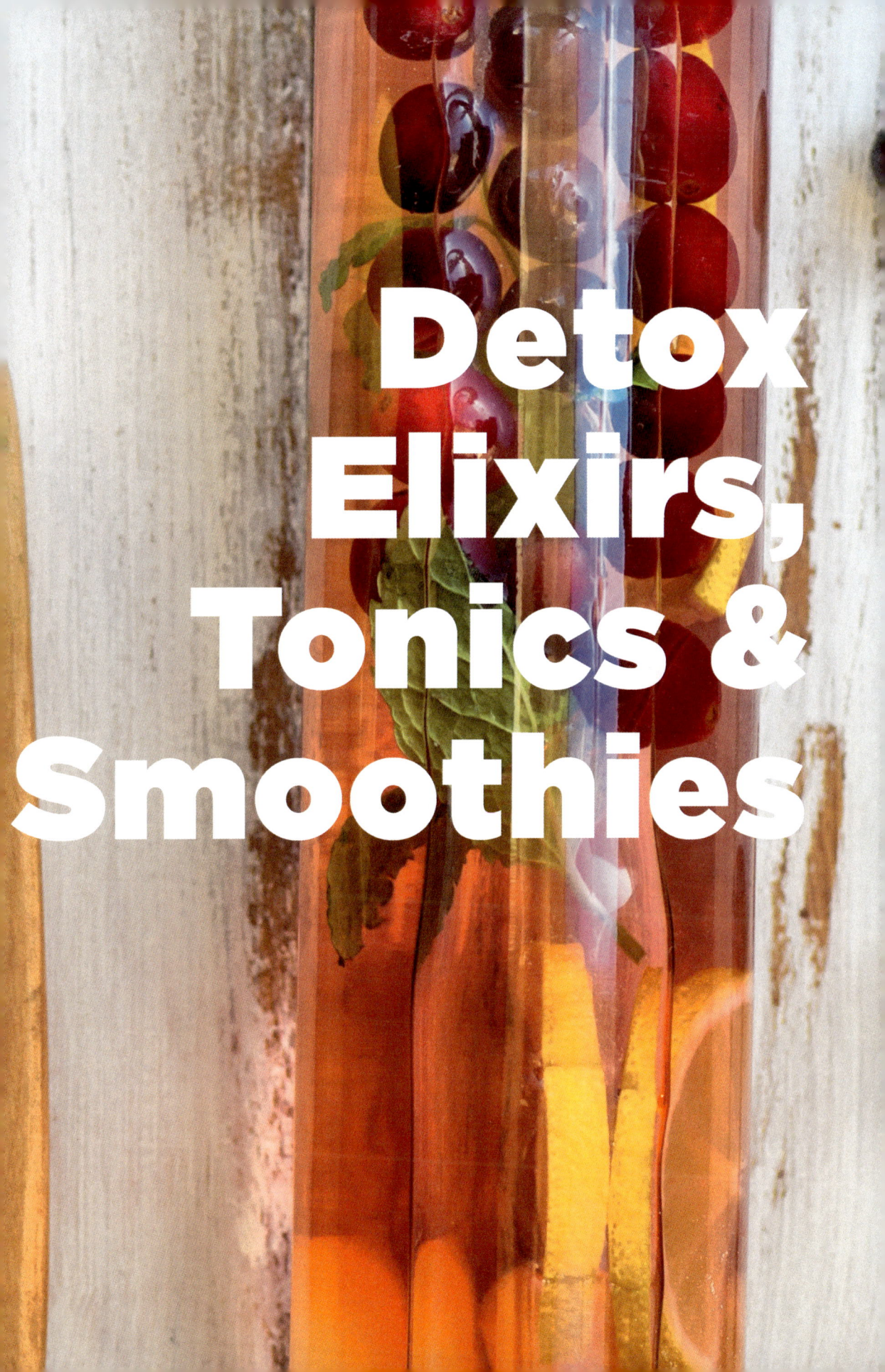

Detox Elixirs, Tonics & Smoothies

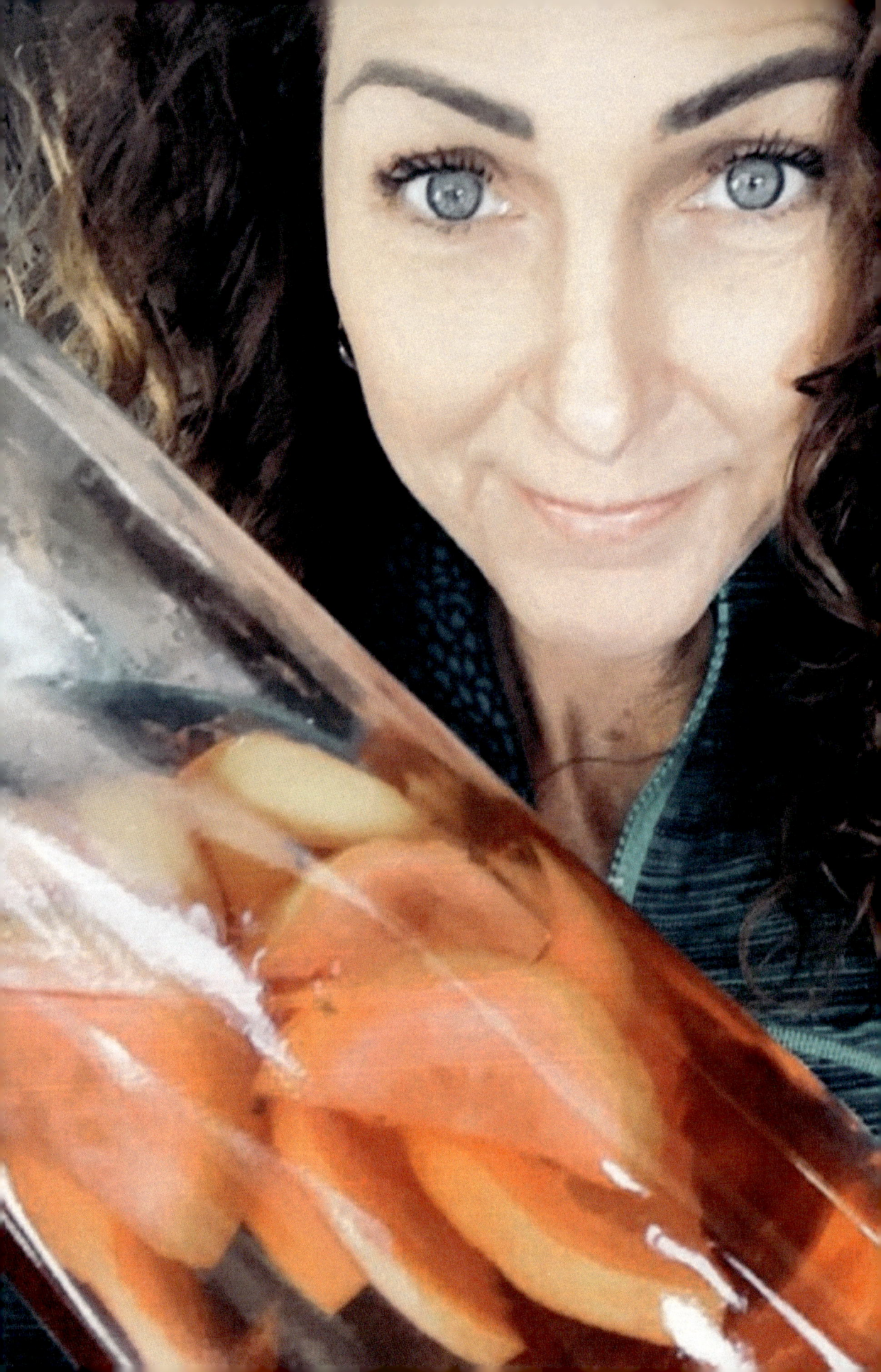

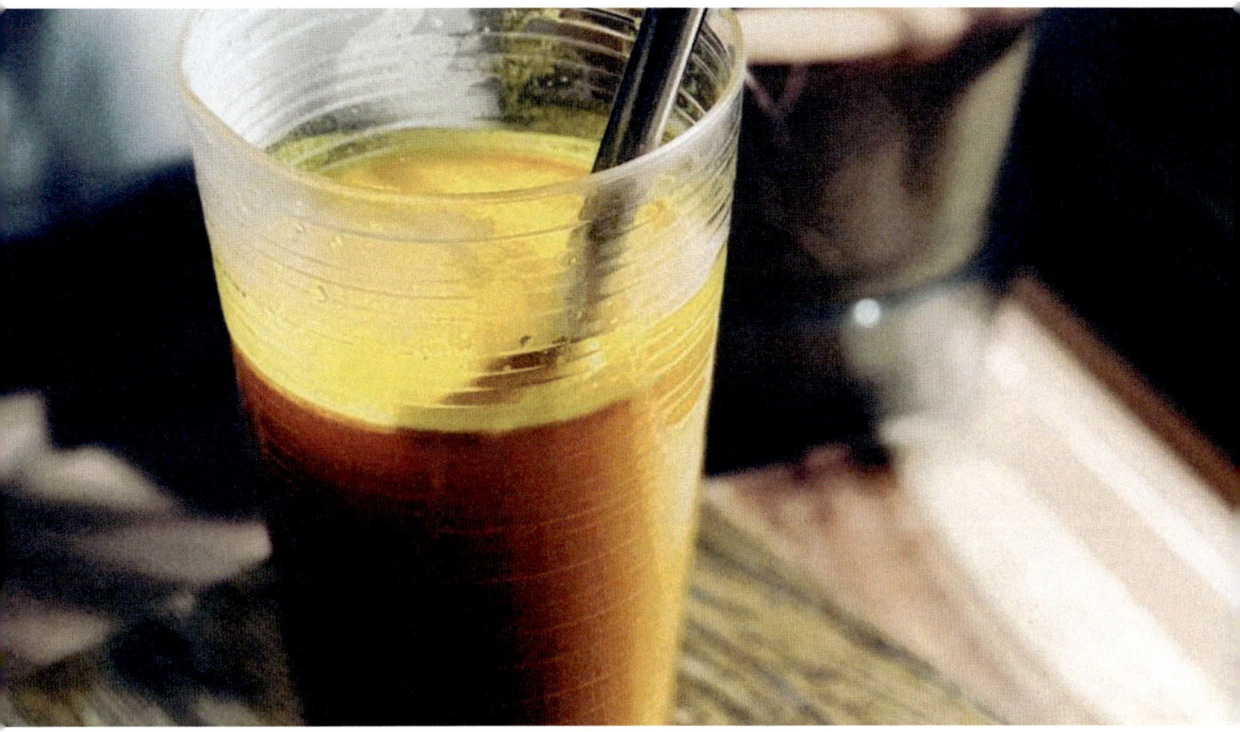

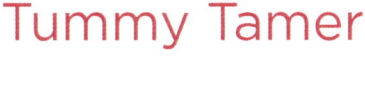

Anti-Inflammatory Brain Booster

1 TBS organic powdered turmeric

Dash of black cracked pepper

1 lemon, juiced

1 TBS ginger juice

Stir into hot water for a warm morning tonic.

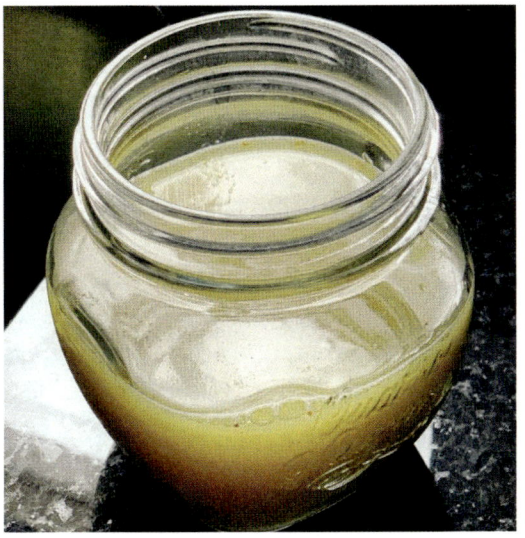

Tummy Tamer

One 2-inch chunk of ginger, peeled

1 ½ TBS fresh lemon juice

2 celery ribs

Blend with water to a frothy warm ginger elixir to soothe your stomach and any inflammation you may be experiencing. Strain if desired.

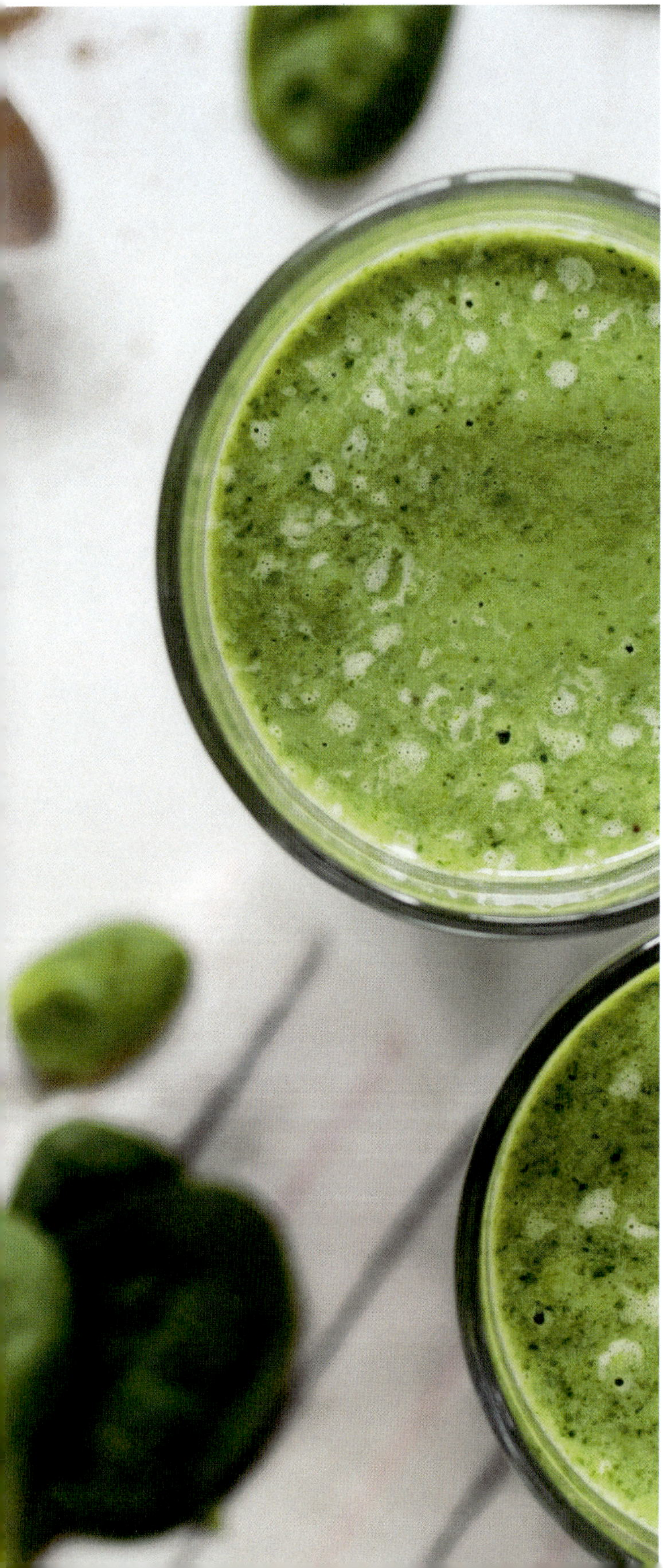

Mango Crush

2 mangos

2 c of baby kale

2 inches ginger, peeled

1 lemon or lime, peeled

1 large handful of sprouts

½ TBS turmeric powder

Add water to achieve desired thickness.

Blend well.

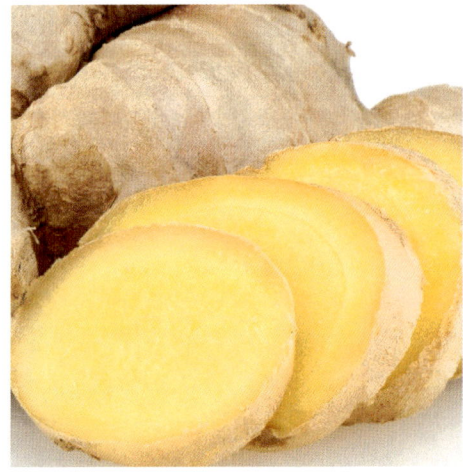

The Clear Cleanser

2 ½ c pineapple

1 banana

2 c of mixed greens

½ c fennel bulb

Add water to achieve desired thickness.

Blend well.

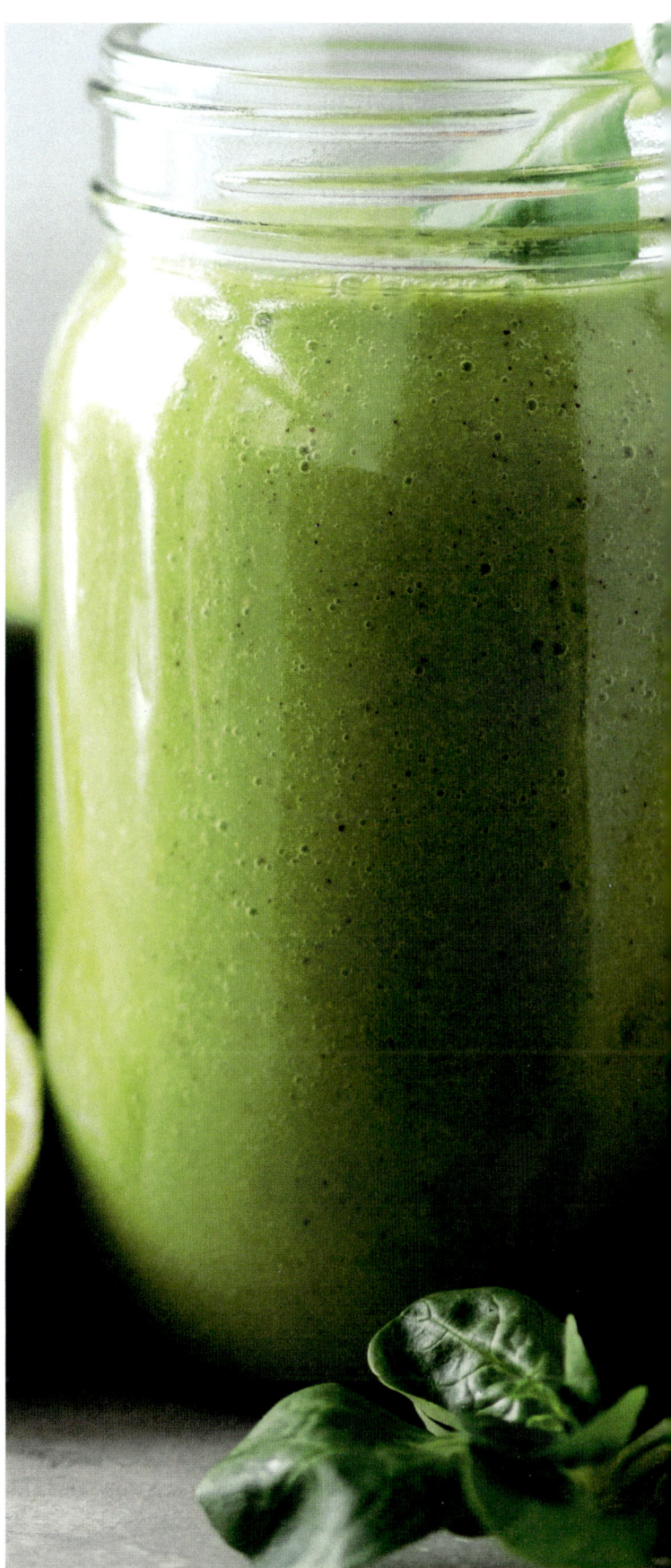

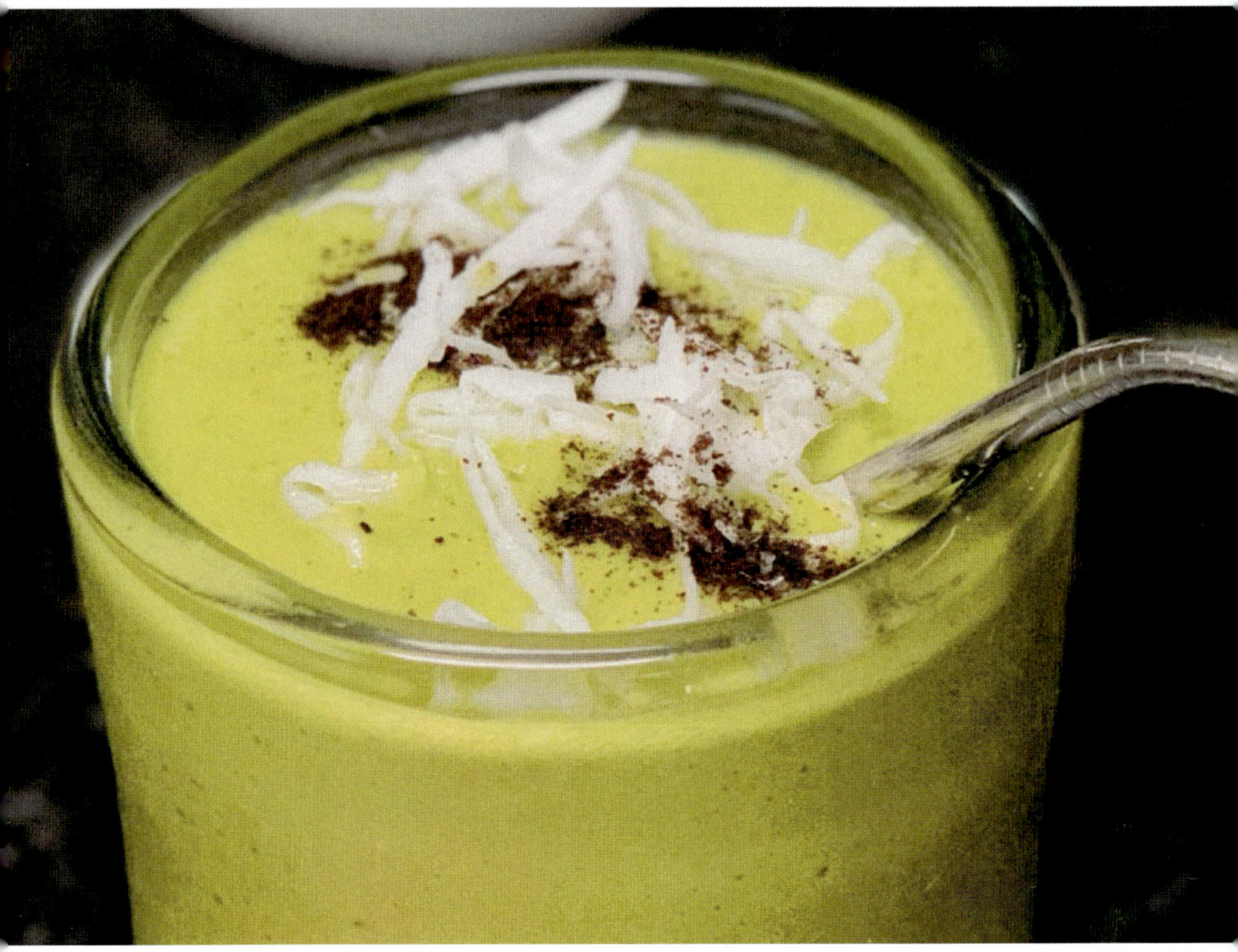

Creamy Coconut Smoothie

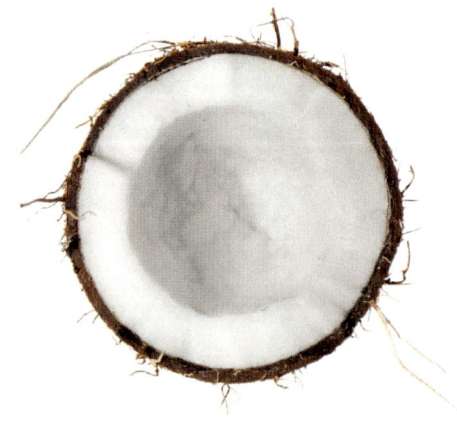

3 frozen bananas

2 c of baby spinach

1 c pineapple

½ tsp vanilla bean powder

1 TBS raw coconut, shredded

Add water to achieve desired thickness.

Blend well.

Vanilla Peach Smoothie

2 peaches, pitted

½ blender full of baby spinach

1 banana

1 TBS chia seeds

1 tsp vanilla bean powder

Add water to achieve desired thickness.

Blend well.

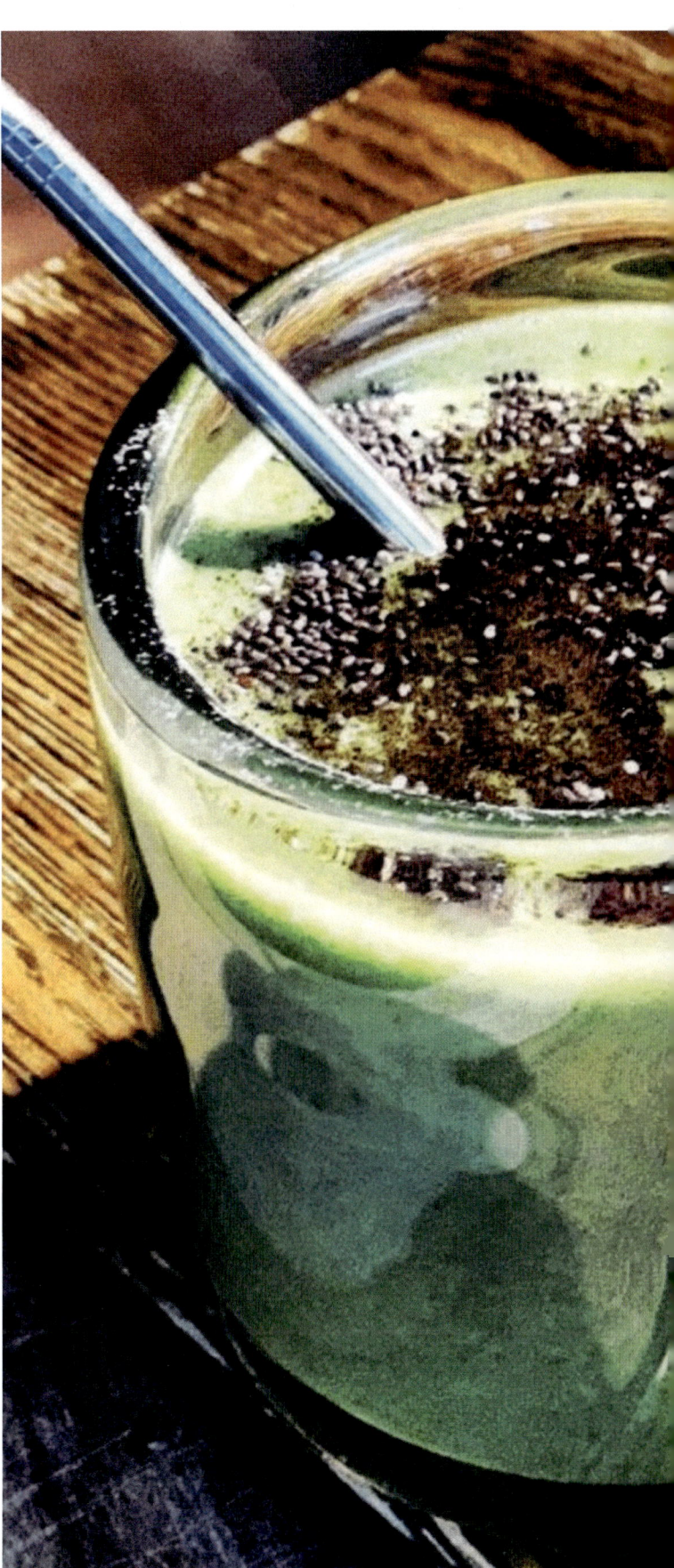

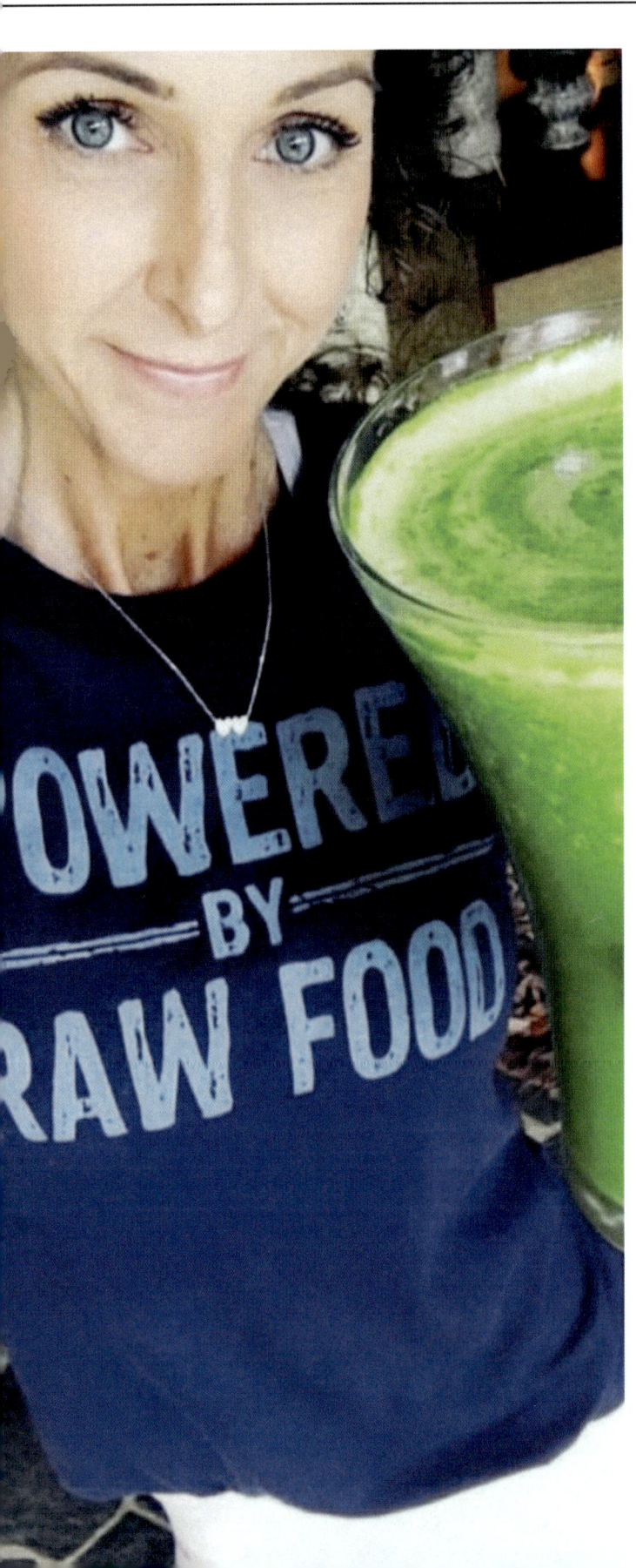

Paradise In A Glass

1 c of coconut water

10 ounces of baby spinach

1 handful of parsley

I lime, juiced

2 c pineapple

1 orange

Add water to achieve desired thickness.

Blend well.

The citrus helps to absorb the iron from spinach and parsley. When I had anemia I drank two of these a day and my iron was back up to normal levels in two weeks. The more greens the better!

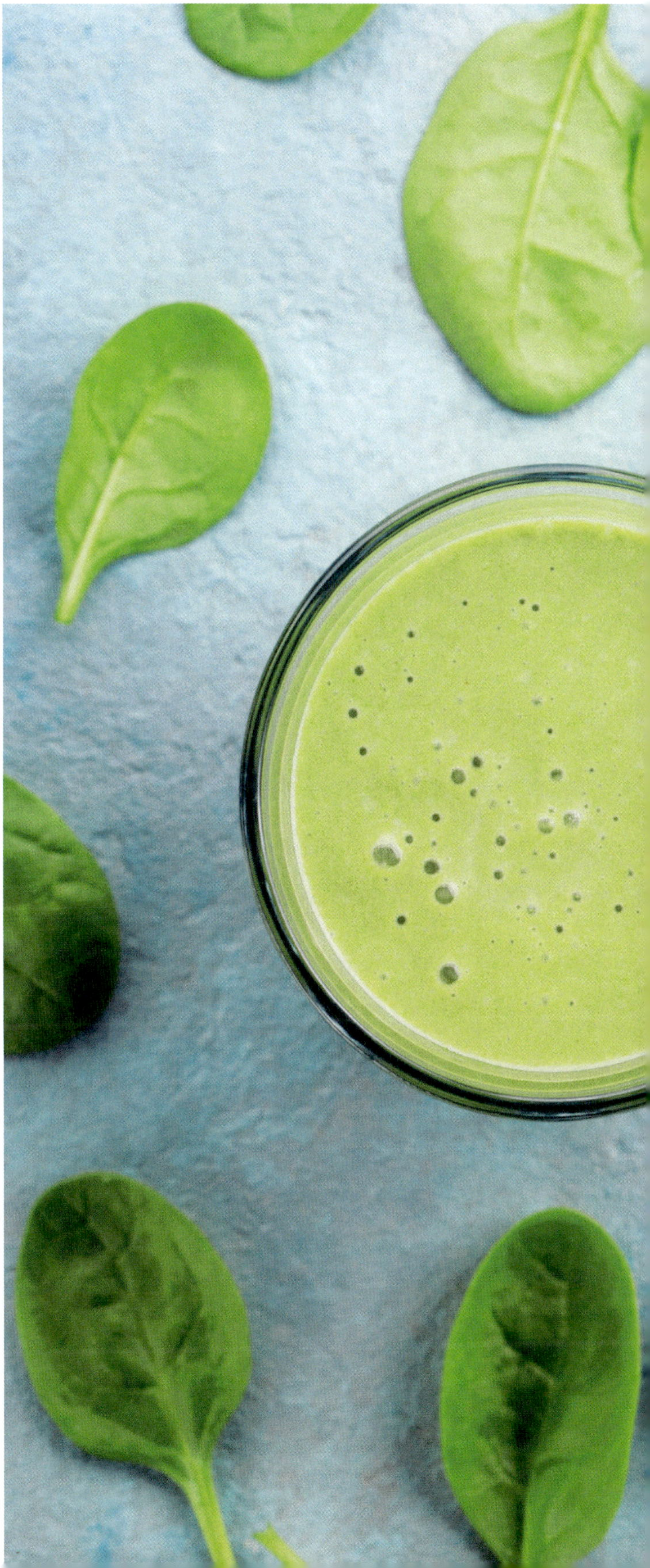

Tropical Storm Smoothie

3 celery stalks

10 ounces baby spinach

1 banana

1 c pineapple

1 inch ginger

Add water to achieve desired thickness.

Blend well.

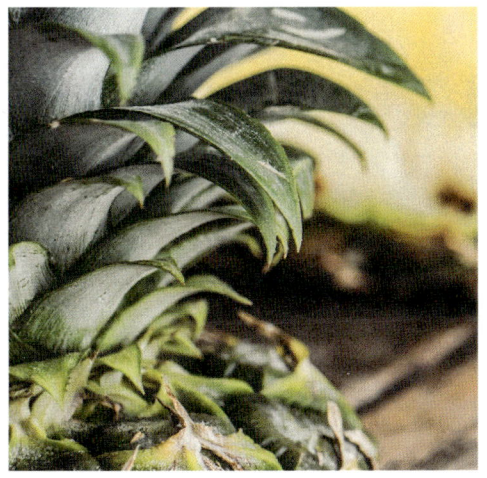

A

Almonds ... 52, 60, 62
Almond Butter ... 47, 54
Anti-Inflammatory Brain Booster ... 71
Apple Cider Vinegar ... 52, 60
Apricots (dried) ... 49
Avocado ... 44, 46, 51
Avocado Dip ... 46

B

Baby Kale ... 72
Baby Spinach ... 74, 75, 76, 77
Bananas ... 73, 74, 75, 77
Banana Peppers ... 51
Blood Orange ... 45
Blood-Orange Butterfly Dressing ... 45

C

Carrots ... 51, 53, 59, 60, 63, 66
Cayenne ... 43, 49, 50, 53, 58, 59
Celery ... 45, 47, 51, 52, 56, 57, 64, 65, 67, 71, 77
Cherry Tomatoes ... 53, 59, 66
Chia Seeds ... 75
Cilantro ... 44
Coconut (Raw, Shredded) ... 58
Coconut Water ... 76
Creamy Coconut Smoothie ... 74
Creamy Pumpkin Seed Dressing ... 56
Cucumber ... 42, 67
Cucumber Avocado Soup ... 67
Cukes & Cream Dipping Sauce ... 42

D

Dates ... 43, 55, 57, 58, 61, 64, 65, 67
Dill ... 44, 52, 65
Dulse Flakes ... 44, 46, 48, 54, 55, 56, 57, 60, 63, 65, 66

E

Easy Peasy Dip ... 50

F

Fennel Bulb ... 64, 73

G

Garlic ... 43, 49, 55, 66, 67
Garlic and Herb Frontier Seasoning ... 48, 50, 54, 56
Garlic Powder ... 51
Ginger ... 51, 67, 72, 77

H

Hearty Carrot Soup ... 51
Hemp-Seed Heart Salad Dressing ... 59
Himalayan Salt ... 52

K

Kelp ... 42, 47, 49, 58, 61, 62, 64

L

Lemon Juice ... 42, 43, 46, 47, 48, 50, 51, 52, 53, 54, 55, 57, 58, 59, 60, 61, 62, 64, 65, 66, 57, 71, 72
Lime ... 76
Lucuma Powder ... 42, 45, 57, 60, 65

M

Mango Crush ... 72
Mangos ... 72
Mexican Fiesta Dip ... 63
Mexican Fiesta Frontier Seasoning ... 45, 63
Mixed Greens ... 73
Mushrooms (Baby Bella) ... 65
My Sweet 'N Smooth Dipping Dressing ... 48

N

Napa Cabbage ... 44, 52
No-Salt Herb Spice Frontier Seasoning ... 67
Nutty Nori Roll Dipping Sauce ... 43

O

On A Coconut Kick ... 58
Orange ... 76
Orange Bell Peppers ... 44, 45, 46, 48, 54

P

Paradise In A Glass ... 76
Parsley ... 76
Peaches ... 75
Peas (raw) ... 50, 64
Peppercorn (Tri-Colored Ground) ... 52
Pineapple ... 73, 74, 76, 77
Pumpkin Seeds (Raw) ... 56

R

Raisins ... 62
Raw Hulled Hemp-Seed Hearts ... 42, 49, 53, 57, 59, 61
Raw Vegan Sauce With A Kick ... 61
Red Bell Peppers ... 44, 46, 47, 48, 54
Red Pepper Flakes ... 52, 60
Roma Tomatoes ... 47, 58

S

Savoury Slaw ... 53
Simple Salsa ... 44
Simple Slaw ... 52
Smoked Paprika ... 51
Smooth & Savory Tomato Dip ... 47
Sprouts ... 72

Sweet Almond Dipping Sauce ... 62
Sweet & Spicy Carrot Almond Dressing ... 60
Sweet Sunshine Carrot and Tomato Soup ... 66
Sweet & Zesty Dipping Sauce/Dressing ... 57

T

Tahini (Raw) ... 48, 49, 53, 55, 59, 63, 64, 66
Tahini Treat Dipping Sauce ... 55
TannyRaw Fennel Pea Soup ... 64
Tanny's So-Simple Sauce ... 54
The Clear Cleanser ... 73
Tomatoes ... 44, 51, 63
Tummy Tamer ... 71
Turmeric (Organic Powdered) ... 71, 72

V

Vanilla Bean Powder ... 74, 75
Vanilla Peach Smoothie ... 75

W

Wakame Seaweed ... 43, 50, 52, 53, 59, 67
Walnut Mushroom Soup ... 65
Walnuts ... 43, 45, 50, 52, 65

Y

Yellow Bell Peppers ... 44, 48, 54, 57, 58, 64
Yellow Squash ... 49, 62
Yummy Yellow Squash Dip ... 49

Z

Zucchini ... 42, 43, 45, 52, 55, 56, 61, 62

Meet Me Online + Take

The Raw Vegan Quiz

How Healthy Is Your Vegan Diet?

Looking for a segue into raw-vegan living but don't know where to start? Maybe you're already raw vegan, but need a little boost of motivation and guidance to keep things interesting.

Get next steps and tips based on your personal results and take your vegan game to the next level.

Go to tannyrawvegan.com

Thank you for your interest in this book!

If you liked this, you'll love these eBooks...

- *Break Free, Butterfly—A 7-Day Raw Vegan Meal Plan Guide*

- *Butterfly Cafe eBook: 77 Raw Vegan Recipes For Transformation*

- *Butterfly Dressings eBook: 45 Raw Vegan Oil Free Salt Free Dressings*

- *Do Different. Get Different. A Journal for Achieving Vibrant Health Through Low Fat Raw Vegan Living*

- *Dressing For Any Occasion eBook*

- *Easy Butterfly Crackers eBook: Foolproof Dehydrating Recipes & Tips*

- *Five-Day Green Smoothie Breakthrough Plan eBook*

- *Fly Butterfly eBook: A Guide To A Successful Raw Vegan Life*

- *Love & Light eBook: 35 Low Fat Raw Vegan Recipes To Get You Through the Winter*

- *Love + Light: A Holiday Meal Guide eBook*

All are available at tannyraw.com.

This book represents the research and ideas of TannyRaw. It is not intended to be a substitute for consultation with a professional healthcare provider before beginning any new diet. The author disclaims responsibility for any adverse effects resulting directly or indirectly from a raw vegan diet.

Made in the USA
Middletown, DE
23 July 2020